The ELIXIR of SPORT

Renew yourself in later life
by playing sports

To Lamb and VAs
You are the elixir of my life

Bike Goddess Press
Copyright 2024 Diana Bartlett. All rights reserved.
ISBN: 979-8-9912572-0-6
Library of Congress Control Number: 2024917949
Cover design by Faisu Graphics

Table of Contents

Chapter 1: Aperitif 7
Chapter 2: ADAP Overview 14
Chapter 3: Deciding to play 23
Chapter 4: Preparing to play 58
Chapter 5: Playing 86
Chapter 6: Benefits of Playing 123
Chapter 7: Discoveries & surprises 147
Chapter 8: Injuries 168
Chapter 9: Not Fifty, but still Nifty 190
Chapter 10: WIIFY? 203
Chapter 11: Resources 229
End Notes 236

Chapter 1
Aperitif

Drink of the elixir and be renewed

What is an elixir? It is a magic potion with the power to bestow renewal, rejuvenation, refreshment to those who imbibe it.

Renewal. Rejuvenation. Refreshment. Those are all "re-" nouns, suggesting that the new, young, and fresh person was inside all along, just awaiting to emerge.

This reinvigorating libation has beguiled humans throughout the ages. The alchemists believed it could perpetuate life indefinitely. In *A Midsummer Night's Dream*, Puck concocts a love-potion that unleases all manner of farce (but all's well that ends well). Some believed an elixir could impart beauty, strength, manliness, and numerous other gifts.

It has appeared in many forms, including magical fountains, questionable herbs, and Botox®!

All cultures revere it.

And, over the millennia, many have pursued it. But, no one has ever managed to capture it.

Until now. This book is about the discovery of an elixir

that's out there at this very moment. It summons no dangerous treks through the jungle, functions without Zeus' intervention, and doesn't require an injection.

This elixir is playing sports in later life.

As the Age-defying Athletes profiled in this volume will demonstrate, you can become renewed by play - even as you enter those illustrious decades that have been variously described as "over the hill", "out to pasture," and "doddering into the sunset".

Aging and improving? Sounds more like a fine wine than an old person. After all, retirees and other aging reprobates conjure up creaky joints, mental fuzziness, and physician groupies.

To repeat: You can renew yourself by playing sports in later life.

Perhaps you are thinking:

"Whoa there, Cowgirl. What a preposterous notion."
Or
"I don't want to look silly..."
Or
"I have no hand-eye coordination, much less foot-eye..."
Or
"I am not competitive..."
Or
"I hated PE..."

Age-defying Athletes voiced similar sentiments. But they overcame all these objections, and you can, too.

To repeat: You can renew yourself by playing sports in later life.

That's the Unique Selling Proposition of this book. To save time, you can stop reading now.

ADAP

The Age-defying Athletes Project (ADAP) captures the stories of real men and women who have drunken that elixir of later life sports play.

The first phase of this Project was interviews with 97 individuals who engage in tennis, golf, pickleball, softball, table tennis, rowing, yoga, and squash. They also swim, ride bicycles, and participate in marathons and triathlons.

As inspiring, not retiring, individuals, ADAP interviewees echo some concepts described by Ken Dychtwald and Robert Morison in their book *What Retirees Want*[1].

One finding from that work is that, now that they have entered retirement, Baby Boomers the world over intend to spend it differently than did their parents. "I want to keep growing and trying new things. I don't want to be as old as my parents were when they were this age," one retiree told the authors.[2]

Being a 70 that's the new 50 is reflected in what retirees want to do with their leisure time.

Dychtwald and Morison discovered that staying healthy/improving health topped the list of retiree leisure priorities, with 83% of respondents selecting it. Relaxing (72%), family connections (58%), fun (57%), and friendships/social connections (56%) rounded out the top five aims.[3]

Age-defying Athletes' initial interest in a sport brought

them to the same starting line as the Dychtwald/Morison interviewees.

But what prompts ADAPers to leap over the starting line? What compels them to return again and again to a sport - even when they lose, play poorly, or describe themselves as having reached their maximum ability? (And even, as Chapter 8 will describe, when they are sidelined with an impairment?)

What powerful nectar is this?

The initial impetus is the promise of a bundle of benefits *a la* Dychtwald and Morison, for sure. Interviewees can articulate these: fitness, fun, friendships, mental health, fresh air, family bonding, and more.

But peel back some layers and it is apparent that the underlying motivational force is self-renewal. These athletes are evolving into better versions of themselves. And they are metamorphosizing even as they age – an all-but-unheard-of phenomenon.

Through playing games, these participants are continuing to grow and develop as human beings. Some may be developing more in the physical realm, some in the psychic, some in externalities like friendship.

As they evolve, they ignore aging stereotypes. Age-defying Athletes continue to attempt things that matter to them, irrespective of how society/well-meaning friends/family members view the wisdom of their actions.

Many interviewees describe one sports benefit along the

lines of "It gets me out there." "Out there" could be out of the house. But it could also mean "out of a rut", "out of what I was yesterday", "out to where life happens".

Self-renewal by playing sports? Really?

Really.

It may be a dramatic renewal, as in the case of Warren[4], who went from being unable to walk due to bad joints to a 30-pound-lighter, swimming version of himself.

Or it could be more subtle. Case in point is 62-year-old Blair, who describes one benefit of tennis as "Committing to doing something – making plans and following through."

Their sense of achievement isn't merely for a better backhand or personal best lap time. The achievement – whatever it is - is their fulfillment. That's the elixir at work.

Fulfillment = self-actualization

Psychologist Abraham Maslow developed the idea of "self-actualization"[5] in the 1940s. He wrote that self-actualization is "self-fulfillment, namely the tendency for [the individual] to become actualized in what he is potentially. This tendency might be phrased as the desire to become more and more what one is, to become everything that one is capable of becoming."[6]

Maslow's idea of self-actualization has been commonly interpreted as realizing one's true potential. (Or, thinking back to the elixir, self-actualization is bringing that new, young, fresh persona forward.)

Self-actualization is a large idea, encompassing the ability to maintain a fresh outlook on life, a desire and capacity to recover from setbacks, an emphasis on the positive, and a continual focus on becoming a better person.

Studies on Masters Athletes have identified a phenomenon similar to self-actualization.

Dr. Rylee Dionigi is a Professor at Charles Sturt University in Australia. Her work with Masters Athletes found that game participation helped them better manage growing older. Subjects reported feeling younger, more vital – in short, more alive.

Some of Dionigi's work is included in a meta-analysis of numerous papers[7] on personal development in Masters Athletes published in 2009.

This analysis noted that "As a result [of their playing Masters Games], the participants expressed a sense of personal empowerment and control over their body and lives that they saw as direct benefits of their involvement in competitive sport. This finding highlights that their sport participation is (in part) a story of resilience, enthusiasm, pride, determination, lives well lived, and lives lived to their potential."[8]

Elixir carried her cross-country

Annie Wilkins

Throughout history, of course, many mature adults didn't really "retire," but went on to do something inspiring.

In 1954, 63-year-old Maine farmer Annie Wilkins rode a horse all the way to California. Her dog came along for the whole trip, too. This astonishing achievement is told in Elizabeth Letts' *The Ride of Her Life, the true Story of a Woman, her Horse, and their Last-chance Journey Across America.*9

The Ride of her Life...the Sports of their Lives. Annie and the ADAP Geezers are inspiring, not retiring. Irrespective of age, gender, athletic resume, sport, skill level, and more, these notable individuals deserve the trophy of renewal.

Let them sip the elixir from that trophy!

They are in it to win it – not just games, but life.

Chapter 2

ADAP Overview

Who are these people?

It's a glorious June morning near a sparkling lake in central Indiana.

Quiet now – eerily quiet, in fact. But not for long. Soon, they would march right in.

First on the courts: a pale couple of indefinite middle age whose last athletic undertaking was racquetball in the 1980s. After retiring, they had decided to try their hands at the fastest-growing sport in America: pickleball. But their serves were undependable, so they always came early to practice before anyone could observe them.

Truck tires crunch on the gravel parking lot adjacent to the courts. A large man with long grey hair tied in a pony tail climbs from the cab. He wears a Big Bend T-shirt, cutoffs, and expensive pickleball shoes.

Another car in the lot, this time a meticulously restored Mustang. When the driver's side door opens, an venerable Janis Joplin tune blares forth. The older guy, a short, shy man in an impeccable yellow polo shirt and matching

Bermuda shorts, says something to the passenger, a younger man in a MAGA hat.

Three bluestockings approach the courts, buzzing softly in conversation punctuated by lots of hand motions. They tote backpacks with paddle handles sticking up. Reaching for the paddles, they hang their packs along the chain link fence.

A stout gentleman with white hair arrives improbably by bicycle. He parks it on the street side of the fence – no locking necessary – and picks up a paddle from the front bike basket. He makes his way onto the court where the three bluestockings have gathered.

A rickety grandmother and her grandson walk slowly toward the courts. Role reversing from the days when she watched him play sports, this time he is observing her, partly to learn the game, partly to be on hand in case she does something to her knees. She had heard pickleball was bad for them.

A grey-haired couple is being walked by two Airedales. They manage to stop the dogs and attach their leashes to the fence. Empty-nesters now, they had read that pickleball was forgiving for bad knees.

The man who owns the biggest house around suffers from chronic back problems. He hunches as he walks and sits down on a bench as soon as he arrives. A minute later, he is up, talking with the pony-tailed guy and the two Mustangers.

Another dog lover is the retired Asian woman who coaxes her Corgi to sit beneath a tree. She never ties him to anything. The woman had heard pickleball was like ping-pong. Even though she had played that as a child, she was never very strong. She hopes the game would help her lose weight.

A Pilates missionary, the neighborhood newcomer is blonde and dressed all in grey. Up close, it is easy to tell that she is probably in her 60s, but from a distance, she appears much younger. Although she looks the part, her shoes aren't right.

An older sedan with heavily tinted windows and racing stripes growls up to the curb alongside the courts and idles. In the front seat, a middle-aged woman opens the door and trades her cowboy boots for sneaks. She wears a blue sweatshirt and has matching blue hair. As the car slithers away, she waves goodbye, walks to a far empty bench and sits down to wait.

Imagine that in just a few minutes, more than 30 people are congregating around six courts. Following playground rules, the later arrivals place their paddles on the right end of other paddles on a rack on the fence. As games are completed, the owner of the left-most paddle hops into the next round.

Men and women over age 50 (some of them well past 50!) of all backgrounds, expectations, skills, preparation, interest, dedication, and energy bounce, hobble, and saunter around the small court.

Why do they do it?

Why would otherwise sane individuals elect to start pickleball 20, 30, or even 40 years since they last swatted a bat or ran cross country? What motivated them to display all their clumsiness and lack of coordination to the world? Why did they risk a dislocated shoulder or pulled groin muscle for the joy of slapping anoversized ping-pong paddle at a whiffle ball?

With all these hurdles, can they really be drinking an elixir of self-renewal? Indeed, they are. Simply by showing up with all their inadequacies and dreams, that's what's happening here in central Indiana.

Even though the Indiana pickleball scene is a composite of many players and several places, it is a realistic scene that tees up the question: Who are these people?

Birth of pickleball

The motley origins of the game may provide some clues about this phenomenon.

According to legend, back in the 1960s, a group of bored Bainbridge Islanders invented the entertainment from what they had on hand – a badminton net, ping-pong paddles, and a whiffle ball.

(Isn't this reminiscent of those 1980s management exercises in which you and your team have to escape from the island on which you are marooned with just a box of paper clips, a wooden spoon, and an HVAC filter?)

Appropriately enough, the game was named – again, per legend – after the "pickle boat" – that is, a vessel crewed by an assortment of individuals who just happened to be around.

People who just happen to be around and are willing to get on board – sounds like most pickleball gatherings which tend toward the informal and loud!

Pickleball is a start-up in the world of established Big Sport. As such, it tends to attract those willing to invest in something novel, to take a risk, to do something, well, almost rebellious. That's part of its appeal.

Then, there is the relative newness of the game. Everyone is, in a sense, a rookie, so the playing field is fairly flat. Another part of the game's appeal.

Plus, it's fun.

The Big Sport Complex

Assorted adults participating in sports, of course, is not limited to pickleball. The Big Sport Complex attracts millions of men and women – many of whom are over age 50.

Specifically in the US:

- Golf - 41 million players with an average oncourse age of 46
- Tennis - 24 million, a third of whom are over age 50
- The great whale of swimming, 91 million participants, where the "50+" box is checked by a third
- Pickleball stats? A puny 9 million today, but with a whopping 86% growth rate over three years. Average age of a "core" player is 48.

The Geezer game community totals in the millions.
But what motivates those millions?

ADAP

In order to discover this, the Age-defying Athletes Project (ADAP) was launched in August 2023.

An ongoing effort, ADAP's first phase was individual interviews with men and women who are never too old to play.

Interview process

Between August 2023-August 2024, 97 individuals were interviewed about their later life sport participation. (Five of these were under age 50 and were analyzed separately; see the "Not Fifty, but Still Nifty" chapter.)

Most total pool respondents (93, or 96%) were interviewed by phone. Four individuals requested in-person conversations. Interviews averaged about 25 minutes in length, although some took almost an hour.

The survey tool consisted of 19 questions aimed at collecting information on when, why, and how interviewees became athletes, and on what the experience has been like.

Over-50 participant details

62 women and 30 men made up this respondent pool.
Their average age was 70, with a range of 51-89.

Over-age-50 details by sport

Sport	Males	Females	Average age (per sport)	Number of interviewees
Tennis	7	27	73	34
Golf	15	24	69	39
Pickleball	2	6	68	8
Marathon	1	1	61	2
Bicycling	1	1	63	2
Swim	1	0	76	1
Triathlon	1	0	71	1
Squash	0	1	58	1
Softball	1	0	70	1
Rowing	0	1	88	1
Ping-pong	1	0	62	1
Yoga	0	1	59	1
Subtotals	30	62		92

Did they come to their current athleticism based on youthful participation? Certainly, over half the pool (54 people) had played one or more sports while growing up, but 38 had not. And 73 had never expected to become athletes as adults.

And even if they had been involved in games as kids, most had lived almost two decades, on average, since taking part in any sport on a regular basis.

The average age at which they began playing their current sport was 50.

Most participants – 79 – were retired, but 13 were still working.

Interviewees fell into three buckets:

• Sports Virgins - men and women who picked up a sport in later life with no prior experience in it

- Prodigals – people who returned to a game after a hiatus of a decade or more
- Continuers – respondents who – more or less - have played a sport most of their adult lives, with no more than a few months' break here and there

This fascinating community of elixir-guzzling Age-defying Athletes will be discussed from numerous angles throughout this book.

Overview of remaining chapters

The Elixir of Sport Chapter 3 considers respondents' beginnings. What was the impetus that pushed Sports Virgins and Prodigals from non-play into (or back into) play? Even the Continuers ...well...continue to make the decision that they will go out and compete. What drives that?

Clearly, all are searching for something to add to their lives. No one mentioned "self-renewal" as the deciding factor, but it was still present in their desires for something novel, something that got them "out there".

Next, Chapter 4 will review how the ADAP community prepared for their sports – everything from formal lessons to do-it-yourself (DIY). Preparation reflected a lot about athletes' personalities as well as about their expectations regarding how difficult or easy a particular game would be to learn and master.

Elixir continues in Chapter 5 with a dive into actual play. That's when Age-defying Athletes really begin to sparkle, to feel that tingle of excitement. Not that they always win – far from it. Most experienced disappointment and frustration. But their power came because they didn't let those factors (permanently) discourage them.

They weren't existentially discouraged because the benefits (Chapter 6) they received outweigh the costs of humiliation, frustration and disappointment. This chapter will explore the rejuvenating benefits Age-defying Athletes enjoyed from playing: fun, fitness (mental and physical), friendships, family, being in the great outdoors breathing fresh air, and more.

ADAPers, as Chapter 7 continues, discovered things about themselves and others, and were surprised by various aspects of their games.

More or less athletic they may be, but they are still Geezers. *The Elixir of Sport's* Chapter 8 discusses how they were injured, how they bounced back, and why they were anxious to return to play as rapidly as possible.

The five under-50 ADAP participants were compared to the larger sample in Chapter 9.

Following that, *Elixir* Chapter 10 features WIIFY? Or What's In It For You?

Finally, Chapter 11 offers a few idiosyncratic resources.
Read on!

Chapter 3

Deciding to play

"You've got to be kidding!"

The glaring morning sun stabbed Dagny's eyes, dividing her visual field – half dark, half light. Balls magically materialized right in front of her.

Dagny squinted, sighed, and regretted that she'd not worn her other hat.

"Focus...focus..."

In return of serve, her partner fired a passing shot against the opposing net player. Ms. Net grabbed it with her strong forehand and shot a steep cross court toward Dagny who just managed to whack it sharply back. The opponent repeated her cross-court zinger, and Dagny responded in kind. Net struck again, but as she did so, began sidestepping back to cover the middle.

"They never expect it three times..." rolled through Dagny's mind. She uncoiled her forehand and slung a crosscourt that narrowly cleared the net. Her opponent tried to recover, but the shot bounced into the alley past her.

Breathing again, Dagny and her partner clicked racquets.

Dagny is 76. Her partner is 69. Their opponents are 49 and 52.

A "super senior" tennis player, Dagny's story illustrates the power of the elixir of sport.

Growing up in a small Iowa town, she learned the game on the two courts at the local high school.

Marriage, kids, career – life interfered and tennis was relegated to an occasional game here and there.

Fast forward 40 years. Dagny has retired, and her work senses finally have disengaged. Even though she long anticipated this "freedom from bondage," now that it's here, she doesn't quite know what to do with herself. She is bored and out of sorts.

Her husband suggests she dust off her old Head® tennis racquet and return to the courts.

"You've got to be kidding," she replies.

"Not at all," he counters. "You always liked it when you used to play."

"I never played very much and certainly don't want to make a fool of myself at my age."

"Well, if you are giving up without even trying, I guess there's nothing more to be said." With that, he left the room.

He knew he had her. She knew he had her.

With trepidation, Dagny signed up for a rookie program at the local tennis club. She was pitiful, swatting an endless stream of shots into the net and out of bounds. To make matters worse, Dagny began to worry about losing her memory - she couldn't recall how to keep score! But she hung on and eventually found her footing.

That was eleven years ago.

Make no mistake. Dagny, competent and steady, is no elite athlete. She is a typical 3.0 player - out there, week in and week out, hitting well, hitting poorly, but always hitting.

She is a composite of several interviewees from the Age-defying Athletes Project, and also reflects findings from the bigger picture of third party research.

The Big Picture

Dagny is not the only retiree who doesn't quite know what to do with herself.

While the 48+ million[10] US retirees dream of how they will enjoy their "golden years," about 21% of them[11] – or 10 million individuals – worry that they will not find meaningful ways to spend their time. In fact, only about 40%[12] of them report pursuing hobbies.

Most retirees are upbeat (Good-bye, tyrannical alarm clock! Sayonara, clogged expressways!). But some of them feel unmotivated and overwhelmed (26%) and are anxious and depressed (24%). 18% worry about "feeling isolated and alone".[13]

Pre-retirees aged 50+ tell a similar tale: 18% worry about finding meaningful ways to spend time; 31% are unmotivated and overwhelmed.[14]

People are looking for something. They need a new lease on life – especially once retirement has demolished the structure they had while working (no matter how much or how little they enjoyed working!).

In short, they need the boost of a sports nectar.

Decision factors motivating ADAPers to play

Men and women searching for something is where the Age-defying Athlete Project begins.

Their perspectives about this search were captured during interviews. One of the key interview discussions revolved around their decisions (a) to play at all, and (b) to play a specific game.

As will be demonstrated throughout this volume, such discussions were keys that unlocked the remainder of ADAP stories – how their "go and play [sport]" decisions led them to a game, and how that game, in turn, brought them the benefits, discoveries, surprises, and, yes, challenges that shaped them into newer, "younger," and better versions of themselves.

ADAP "Why play?" overview

A scan of ADAP research identifies several interesting answers to "Why play at all, and why pick that particular sport?"

First, reasons why echo some of the Dychtwald and Morison findings mentioned in Chapter 1.

For example, Age-defying Athletes wanted a hobby, they desired to do something to fill their retirement years, and the like.

And, similarly with the Dychtwald/Morison interviewees, ADAPers sought something more than merely a method for whiling away the hours.

That "more" encompassed friendship, fitness, and fun as the stated rationale for ignoring aches and pains, feelings of inadequacy, lack of talent, and more so that they could... well...just go out and play.

Second, despite the straightforward "friendship, fitness, and fun" reasons driving their sport choices, their actual sport selection was more of a "package" that mixed together the respondent's life stage, influencers, interest in a particular game, anticipated benefits, skill self-perception, and more. To pick a sport, Age-defying Athletes used a matrix of reasons rather than a simple ranking of athletic pursuits.

If a man or woman elected to "get fit," for instance, he or she rolled that decision up with factors such as perceived skill, game availability, existing fitness level, curiosity, schedule, plain old-fashioned interest, and more. That's how a pickleball or swimming selection came to be.

Third, keep in mind that these participants described the same decision factors using different terms. For example, some may have listed "camaraderie" as the reason they decided to play, while others explained that they wanted to "meet people" in a new town.

Fourth, many respondents noted more than one factor behind selecting, say, running or bicycling. One marathoner, for instance, reported that he began by a desire to get fit, but that he also wanted to support his kids on a camping trip.

Details about the sport selection decision

Because of the above variability, the following summary gathers decision reasons into loosely defined categories whose boundaries are subject to ebb and flow.

These choice categories are applicable for Sports Virgins, Prodigals, and Continuers. No apparent decision factor trend distinguished any of the three.

Perhaps most important, decision factors also turn up as benefits once play begins. It's not that often in human endeavors that the goal one initially sought is actually achieved! But with that elixir of sport, it happens.

Friendship, including family

Almost two-thirds of the reasons that respondents elected to play a game were people-related:

- Camaraderie
- Friendship
- Meet people, especially after moving to new community
- Spouse influence, frequently spouse influence paired with retirement
- Work related – including colleagues who encourage getting involved
- Kids - sons, daughter, kids gone, son sent pickleball set to their summer home
- University roommate

- Brother-in-law left golf clubs in his garage
- Love

Fitness

This factor amounted to about 10% of the decision drivers:

- Lose weight
- Sharpen thinking
- Fresh air and walking

Fun

Fun is a capacious decision category:

- Joining a club/discounted club membership equated to 7% of the rationales
- For fun and "as a lark" drove 5% of respondents to their respective sports
- Another 4% were focused on the games themselves and "always loved it" (a Prodigal tennis player) or wanted to become serious and to improve their playing
- Wanted a "hobby"

A mixed salad of other decision drivers

4% started due to factors only indirectly related to the sport:

- One pickleballer faced the loss of racquetball courts and had to transition to the new game
- One woman took up bicycling simply as a way to strengthen her legs for a 100 mile hike with her husband
- Another cyclist needed transportation around a small town and that's why he adopted bicycling

And, finally...

- Two respondents "fell into it"
- One golfer said that her husband convinced her to do it because golf was the only game that allowed drinking and smoking while playing (See below for Langley's story.)
- A female pickleball enthusiast adopted the sport after a tennis injury sidelined her from that game
- One was seeking something "novel" to do
- A tennis player stated the game was the only thing for which he had time back in the day when he was still working
- Perhaps most revealing of all, a 62-year-old who had just begun golfing three years ago wanted "rejuvenation"

(Decision reasons total more than 100% due to multiple reasons for numerous interviewees.)

ADAPer stories

Here are a few real-life ADAPer stories that illustrate how a taste of the sports brew motivated them to jump (or be dragged) into a game. These stories will also provide a peek at how their decisions turned out.

Motivated by Friendship

Belinda

When asked how old she is, Belinda responds that she is 86, but that she prefers the expression "climbing the aging ladder" instead of "aging".
"Attitude is vital."
Did she play sports while growing up? "I grew up in rural Montana so nothing was available to a girl in the 1940s."
"Tennis was never a part of anything I could do."
Even though she ran for 25 years, Belinda did not participate in any contact sports.
Fast forward four decades and Belinda was nearing retirement. Her nieces in Mississippi encouraged her to visit and see the Gulf Coast. It was certainly a change from Montana – especially in February!
Upon her return to The Treasure State, Belinda began to plan her move south, which she did the following year.
Over about the next four-year period, she bought a tiny house near the Gulf and created a gorgeous garden in her back yard.

But all the while, she was considering the game. "I began [playing tennis] sporadically."

Eventually, she played more consistently. "I was prompted because I knew no one [in the new community] except my nieces and I thought I couldn't make a life based on them. Then I joined a local tennis club and started lessons with a pro there, and that's how I met my tennis group."

To Belinda, the most difficult aspect of learning was "my confidence level. Am I too old? But life is a new adventure."

"I had gone to a retirement workshop while I was still working" she relates, "and the speaker told us life has three phases: go-go, slow-go, and no-go. So, I became very focused on prevention and the importance of activity."

Belinda has since discovered that taking up tennis has increased her confidence. "As my Mom used to say, '*Can't* can't do anything.'"

Besides building friendships and boosting her confidence, tennis has delivered other benefits. "My doctor says she cannot believe that I am doing all I do at my age. Tennis has helped my thinking and health, keeps me socially active, and it's good for hand-eye coordination. If I'm not playing, I walk three to five miles."

Tennis is surprisingly difficult, according to Belinda. "Not just a matter of hitting a ball – but coordination and movement. Constantly improving is important. I want my movement and strokes to improve and be more graceful. I can feel my brain and feet talking to each other! I also want to develop strategy."

"I am motivated by positive feedback from friends and

playing partners," Belinda reveals. "...Also motivated by the improvement in my game."

She attends drills sometimes, to hone her net skills, her serve and return.

"Sometimes, I will go to a court by myself and practice serves."

Four years ago, Belinda was walking back to her home and tripped on a sidewalk that had been damaged in a recent storm. "I fell and broke my left elbow. A plate was implanted and I was out for three months, then four more months of PT [physical therapy]. During that time, I walked up to seven miles a day to keep my muscles tuned and my stamina, high."

Motivated by Love

Borden

When interviewed, Borden was a 71-year-old retired electronics company executive in the Midwest. Even though he took up golf in his late 20s, "I didn't think of golf as a sport."

But, as he revealed in his story, he had met a woman who would become his wife, and says that "We dated. She was avid [about the game]. So what the heck?"

Borden continued with this love story – love for a woman and love for a game: "I went to the driving range with her, using old clubs." She also took him to par three courses.

"I was hooked after the first summer...by the second summer, I started lessons and joined a country club."

Golf eventually overtook some pre-existing athletic passions. "At the time," Borden recalled, "I played basketball, baseball, and was at the height of my tennis playing."

Sports were "a major theme in my life. Baseball, basketball from young age, influenced by my Dad. Starting in junior high, played tennis through my 20s. Picked up tennis again in my 50 and 60s. No college sports, only intramurals.

"I bowled 10 to 15 years when it was popular and achieved a certain level of performance."

His father had had ambitions for him to play at a high level, although not necessarily at a pro level.

"In high school, however, I realized that athletics were not my future."

Nonetheless, he remained active in at least one sport for the rest of his life.

"I love watching high level sports, and want to play at a comfortable high level," stated Borden. "I enjoy sport for enjoyment sake. I love playing sports, going to play is a privilege and [I] layer benefits on that. I will overcome barriers to play golf...it's attractive and joyful."

Given this intense athletic environment, it's not surprising that Borden married an athletic woman. "My wife ... came from a golfing family."

He described her as "an incredible advocate and mentor for the game of golf. My biggest cheerleader in the exploration of [the game]."

Her support, Borden continued, was vastly important.

However, the golf gods can be capricious, and Borden encountered challenges with the links.

"The difficulty [with golf]," he noted at the time, "was

getting to a level of performance I was satisfied with. The ball is just sitting there. I picked up sports quickly, but not golf. That was frustrating.

"I thought it wouldn't be hard to become a scratch golfer," he continued, "but the best I ever achieved was a nine handicap. Really thought I could be better. Commitment? Skill?"

Still, Borden pronounced golf a great game. "...can play entire life. Find joy in playing, great excuse to be socially active, walk through beautiful nature, so many interesting people."

Borden had been playing twice a week, and his goal was "Today, have fun. If not [having] fun, missed the whole thing. Meet interesting people."

Golf had also taught him humility. "I was a successful career person, but when I play golf, regardless of success in life, success is not guaranteed."

This accomplished and happy man, unfortunately, had to exclude himself from the game for many months.

"I was away from golf two years fighting cancer and returned to golf, but the game today is quite different than it was three or four years ago," Borden states. "Blessed that I can play again. Shocked how much I lost physically."

He continued: "I should practice, but I don't and not sure why. Attitude and schedule [probably]. I could work out more and [that's] something I need to try to understand. Three to four workouts a week pre-cancer."

He also used to practice pitch shots and drives before his illness.

In the final analysis, golf had been a significantly positive force in Borden's life.

He listed some of the benefits he's received from the links: "Social aspects – guy friends, couples. Great to play with wife. Cornerstone of our social life. Every club which we have joined enabled this except [one overseas club where they were expats]."

Motivated by Fun

Langley

"Golf is the only sport that encourages smoking and drinking at the same time [as playing]."

So Langley, 62, was told by her husband who had started playing golf as an adult. It was a compelling argument for fun.

"I had played tennis for about ten years before taking up golf [at age 50]," the Floridian explains. "[My husband's] parents were big tennis players, but tennis took a toll and I was fatigued by it."

Even though as an adult she was a "heavy sport user," the most athletic thing Langley had done while growing up was cheerleading.

"I was never athletic," she claims. "I had three sisters, Dad was in the military, money was tight, and my parents wouldn't do anything for one sister that wasn't done for all, so [sports were] too expensive for all four girls."

Langley began golf with lessons at the driving range. "I got a starter set of clubs for Christmas and took six to ten lessons on the mat at the range."

At first, she only wanted to play with her husband on weekends at 4PM so no other golfers would follow them. "I didn't want anyone to see me playing."

Not only did she not want to be seen on the course, but she wouldn't play with anyone except her husband. If additional names were on the tee sheet, she refused to play. "Eventually, I got used to being with other golfers. Pace of play is more important than how you play."

Golf has turned into a great experience, Langley says. "I have 28- and 32- year-old daughters and so now when they visit, we play together and then play in Indianapolis where they live. Husband plus me plus now daughters. Surprising thing is how I can play in this heat and in cold weather, too."

Like Belinda, Langley cites confidence as a sport fact of life. "I like competition and like to play with people who are not better than I am. That builds my confidence. Better players get into my head."

Still, she plays respectably, and even won a nine-hole Ladies Golf Association (LGA) tournament. "My goal is to consistently score below 100. I'm now at around 106-108, occasionally 102."

Despite her dedication to golf's fun side, socialization is also motivating. "We are a stay-at-home couple, so golf is the main reason we go out."

Motivated by fitness

Reynaldo

Reynaldo's parents had moved to the US from Argentina. As a result, organized school sports were "not a big thing. My parents were immigrants and when I was growing up, it was all about school."

Nonetheless, Reynaldo enjoyed informal playground games such as basketball and softball. "I did not do track and field."

And at age eight, he dreamed of playing center field for the Yankees.

Today, however, Reynaldo – who describes his age as "in my 60s" - doesn't consider himself an athlete, even though he has achieved some significant athletic accomplishments.

Reynaldo also excelled academically, and earned a PhD. He pursued a career in the aerospace industry, married, and then welcomed two sons into the world.

Throughout this period, there was no time for sports.

"Into my 30s," he recalls, "there were things like company softball and I would occasionally play. In my 40s, I ended up coaching my kids in baseball and basketball because I loved the sports."

Reynaldo notes that "Our kids ended up loving them, too. My older son played water polo and baseball, and my younger was on basketball teams through varsity level."

Kids became his athletic "outlet". Thus, it's no surprise that when Reynaldo was in his late 40s, he relished the chance to join his sons for a two-week Boy Scout outing in Colorado.

"The elevation was ten to twelve thousand feet, so everyone had to be in shape. I decided to start running with my boys, but couldn't even run a block before I started choking and spitting."

Those decades without sports had taken a toll. "I realized how quick and easy it was to fall out of shape."

He continues: "Fortunately, I had two to three months to get in shape and worked up to a three-mile run. I also lost 20 pounds. We made the trip successfully."

When they returned, "I realized I was in the best shape of my life and said it would be a shame to fall out of fitness again."

Unlike most other ADAP respondents, Reynaldo investigated other sports as a way to stay fit. He discovered that "basketball, which I love, was probably not a good idea for a middle-aged man."

But there was always running, which had worked well for that mountain trip. Some of his co-workers ran 10Ks and half marathons and they encouraged him to try those. "I started doing 5Ks, then within about a year and a half, ran a half marathon."

There was social encouragement, but Reynaldo is a self-described introvert and didn't join any running club. "I like to do things on my own."

But he did have one-to-one conversations with some at his workplace. "They recommended a couple of books, including Galloway's *Run-Walk-Run Method*[15].

"The book prescribes starting at your own running ability to avoid discouragement," Reynaldo explains. "You run one minute, walk one minute, and then after a while, increase the run to two minutes, with the one-minute walk, and work up to five minutes' of running with a one-minute walk. A five-minute run is almost a mile, so then you're on your way.

"I live in a wonderful neighborhood for running, but because I was a little intimidated by cars, I would run four times around my block at night. I worked up from there."

He reports that after completing a half marathon, "I thought, 'Why not do a full marathon?' After all, I was in the best shape of my life, even better than when I was in high school."

Reynaldo captures the essence of the elixir when he says, "I felt on top of the world, even if I was older. I could age and stay in shape. Because of all the miles I've put in and my physical shape at [my] age, [it] enables me to perform well. I have developed a fitness commitment and habit of life."

He discovered that he had something in common with sport greats. "Not that I could play basketball like Michael Jordan, rather than like the gym rat that I am," he declares. "But it's that I have accomplished something worth achieving, something that I didn't think I could do, and that not many people have done. Whether fast or slow, there is this sense of achievement, knowing what I had to put myself through to get there."

Over the last ten or so years, Reynaldo has completed more than a dozen marathons. He loves the fact that he can go on a vacation or business trip and just run wherever he is.

And despite the fact that this story began with a health-related need, his prime motivation today is the next race or destination. "Good health is not enough," he states.

"I need the discipline of a race, of a deadline. Otherwise, I would never train."

These days, he typically participates in one marathon annually, possibly two.

Reynaldo says that traveling internationally to marathons is a great way to persuade his wife to accompany him.

Reynaldo came around to superb fitness after starting with the intention of bonding with his sons.

Motivated by other decision drivers

Work, work, work

Like Reynaldo, a couple of Age-defying Athletes backed into a sport due to work-related circumstances.

One woman who heads a not-for-profit organization, for example, had joined a dining club in order to have a good place to take clients for lunch.

Subsequently, she discovered that the club also featured squash courts. Although she had last played squash 30 years prior – in undergraduate school - she soon was back in the game. Having an active ladies' program was a definite plus.

Another woman began a late-life golf career because all the other accountants in her CPA firm would periodically disappear for a day on the links. She decided that sounded good to her and tagged along.

A racqueteer previously had been a dedicated basketball player. But a job transfer landed him in a new location that offered no basketball at lunchtime.

However, there were industry events around tennis, especially doubles, and there was a lot of camaraderie. So he switched to another type of "court".

Veronica

A more serendipitous work-related occurrence was the deciding factor for Veronica, 88.

To start at the start: Veronica grew up (and has lived most of her life) in a mid-sized city that is home to one of the largest public universities in the south.

"...when I was young ...ages six through nine... I just played softball with boys in our neighborhood during softball season. And then when it was football season, I played touch football with them. Same thing for basketball in season.

"Swimming, too. I participated in city league girls swim races," Veronica continues. "I was short, always about an inch behind the taller girl who always won. We became great friends and still are."

Despite this all-round sports involvement, she never expected to become an athlete. "There wasn't such a thing for girls. No girls competititions except church league - in which I played girls softball."

Coming from modest circumstances, Veronica was able to attend the university because, in her freshman year, the first semester tuition was $25.

She lived at home to save the dorm fee. Her Mom and she shared the family car.

Always interested in the scientific study of human body movement, Veronica earned a PhD in kinesiology from the university. She went on to build and eventually lead an international kinesiology research and education department at the school.

Always active, Veronica was a runner for many years, and also took up golf.

However, when she was 60, she fell in love with rowing.

"It was because of a grad student who was an exercise physiologist who had the lab right across the hall from my office," she relates.

"We were good friends. He reviewed my book, [on the physical dimensions of aging] and commented that its big flaw was that it contained no reference to rowing."

The student introduced her to the ergometer – also known as a rowing machine. "I used that four or five times and liked the way it felt. I asked him to teach me on water, but he said go to [the local] Rowing Club for lessons because 'I'm too busy!'"

The Club participated in national learn-to-row day, as well as provided instructions.

But Club instruction wasn't ideal.

Veronica describes the environment then: "These were early classes and they put coxswains not well trained in boats. Sometimes coxswain didn't show up, so we couldn't go out. One cursed and I didn't respect her."

To make matters worse, one of the new instructors was "bad".

"I hesitated a little [about continuing]," Veronica says. "But fortunately, a woman from England was in charge –

Charles River crew and an excellent coach. She ensured that every person got into a boat. Her teaching was very good."

As a result, she continues, "I fell in love with it. Loved being on the lake. I dropped my golf for rowing – golf took too much time and I was always angry afterwards..."

She had also been running for a long time, and abandoned that for rowing, too.

Veronica was 60 when she first picked up oars, and has been rowing for 28 years.

When asked to describe the experience of rowing, Veronica begins her response in true scientist fashion:

"There's always something in the sky that's really interesting – clouds, birds, helicopters. Some trees contain hundreds of birds. We go out early and sometimes see the sentinel birds awakening – they are used to our boats. The rest of the birds wake up and fly horizontally and never run into each other. Turtles on logs. Fishermen on banks."

She adds that she "..really likes the way I feel when I get off the water, even in heat and humidity. Not true with golf."

In the Club, the more competitive rowers go out earlier than she typically does. They're in the water at 5:45A until about 7. "We start later and row for about an hour-and-a-half."

Veronica rows in a double boat – two oarsmen, each with two oars.

"I'm the one that sets the rate in rowing. My friend and I both face backwards, but because she's in the bow, she has to turn around to see where we are going.

"I also row in an eight. That's a co-ed boat, four men and four women. To balance the weight, men and women are interspaced."

Rowers are always taking lessons. When they're in the water, Veronica notes, "Patrol boats with coaches come up on rowers and coach strokes, usually every time we go out."

Coaching is important because the sport combines both power and precision.

"The difference between rowing double and rowing an eight [was surprising]," Veronica explains. "In the eight boat, we are trying to synchronize two oars on each of eight people by the coxswain. In and out of water same time and we sometimes [manage to] do that."

And sometimes not...

Her goal is "always trying to perfect the stroke and make it easier to row better."

She and her crew mates are preparing for the fall regatta in the eight boat. "Doing drills – fast take off and work on force for each stroke and perfect synchronization. Legs do all the work, arms just keep oars in position."

Veronica says that she is "...more motivated to row than not." Perhaps that's why she adds that "I'm a fanatic about something which has surprised me. And I can make myself work hard."

That hard work includes three days per week of "practice" on her home ergometer.

Additionally, she's in the water four times weekly, if the weather is decent, with no rain. "If it's really windy," she expands, "we cannot go out because the double [boat] sits low in the water."

Her four "water" days are the double boat Monday and Friday, the eight on Wednesday and Saturday

Days of the week make a difference.

"Saturdays," reports Veronica, "everyone is on the water, but we go down to the dam, where there aren't many stand-up paddleboarders. Those [paddleboards] are mostly rented and the users hang around the rental place more toward town."

"I rest on Sunday."

The key benefit for Veronica? "I've been able to row and locomote very easily to my current age, 88. I attribute this to rowing, and that was a good shift away from running."

Rowing Club members pay monthly dues. "That lets you row anything in the boat house for which you are skilled – novice, middle (mid), advanced,"

Veronica says that "Novice boats are wider and better balanced. Mids, narrower. Advanced, even narrower and less stable, but faster.

"I use club oars, too – also novice, mids, advanced."

Veronica is a lifelong athlete of amazing performance. However, this didn't keep her from injury. And this occurred not while she was in a boat on the water, but, oddly enough, at her home.

As she tells it, she became dizzy and passed out at her house a couple of months ago. This caused her to fall down her stairway.

Veronica was in the emergency room from 8:30A until 10:30P that day. The hospital insisted on keeping her for three days. "They were scared to death I would do it [pass out] again."

No bones were broken in this fall, fortunately. However,

she adds that "Afterward, I couldn't use my right arm well because of skin loss from fall. Very painful. Couldn't move elbow. Just waited it out."

Injury

And that's an appropriate lead-in to the next category of decision driver: injury. One female tennis player had experienced a serious impairment to her elbow and decided to seek a less rigorous alternative in pickleball.

Boredom

As Dychtwald and Morison touch upon in their research, boredom can be a powerful motivator.

"When I was 35 or 40," relates Felicity, "we lived in a neighborhood that had tennis courts and a swimming pool. There wasn't much else around, so we all went down [to the courts] and I played some…"

Facility closure

It was by process of elimination that Sam moved from racquetball to pickleball. He had played the former game for several years, but faced a dilemma when the racquetball courts were eliminated in favor of pickleball ones during a gym renovation. "Pickleball, here we come!"

Transportation

Process of elimination also contributed to Hans' decision to settle on cycling as a way to solve a pragmatic problem.

A few years back, he was approached about a new job. It would be a terrific position, one for which his strong analytical skills would be well suited. The organization was prestigious, unique in Denmark. Excellent pay, smart colleagues, advancement opportunities galore.

Terrific job opportunity except for one thing – it was almost 200 kilometers from his home. And his family did not want to relocate.

Hans took the job anyway, opting for a small, cheap flat near the office. He would live there during the week, and then spend weekends with his family.

"[Deciding to cycle] was just a coincidence. I needed a bike for transportation, so I was just looking at this pragmatically. Off the shelf bikes were more expensive than I recalled. So, I searched for second-hand bikes for one that was similar to one I used when I was a kid. But these required repair."

Hans relates that he "...started to fiddle around with bikes, functioning more like a bicycle shop. I did not road race. I enjoy dealing with mechanical parts.

"Once a bicycle had been repaired or refitted, I would ride it to test it, and that's how I got back into bicycling."

An unexpected thing happened when he took the bike out for a test ride. He actually enjoyed the ride for its own sake – not simply as a way to get around, but as a method of clearing his mind and feeling himself move through space.

"[I] just started biking. It was easier than playing soccer! I had been off and on with soccer in recent years.

"Actually, when I started the mechanic side," he asserts, "it took a lot of energy. It was more like when I was younger and tinkered with our kids' bikes."

Hans makes fascinating connections: "I can interpret physics and math via bike mechanics. Amazing how well-designed bikes, bearings, fittings, and the rest are. I can see the 'physics' of bicycles. This is unlike my professional work as a physicist, in which I analyze particles far too small to see or otherwise perceive."

Perhaps unexpectedly, he is "...better with my work which involves theoretical thinking. My equations are more productive.

"A great discovery has been to learn the joy of working with things. It's mindless and mindful simultaneously."

There were unanticipated health advantages, too. "Something that surprised me in all this is that I lost weight from cycling," Hans claims. "My MD had said I needed to lighten up for 20 years. But all my prior efforts [e.g., swimming], were unsuccessful. But as soon as I started cycling, I lost weight."

"What's more, I sleep well," Hans notes with pride. "I previously had high blood pressure, now blood circulating better. No aches and pains. Back is stronger and joints healthy."

Fell into it

The old saying is that not to decide is to decide. In like fashion, some ADAP interviewees "made" a non-decision, and they just "fell into" a sport.

Winston, 71, and Cora, in her 60s, for example, "fell into" triathlons – and went on to participate in them for several years. (More about Winston and Cora in Chapter 4.)

Factors that <u>failed</u> to motivate a sports decision

Thus far, this chapter has discussed friendship, fitness, fun and a couple of other variables that exerted a tractor beam pull toward a sport.

There are three other motivators that also should have exerted that pull but which, for one reason or another, did not.

The first of these is online sport-matching sites, which will be expanded on, below.

The second and third ones relate to childhood experiences with games. As will be shown, lack of experience did not weigh heavily on the choices to play in the first place nor on which sport to play.

And rich athletic experience – leading in a couple of cases to Olympic tracks – didn't directly translate to later athletic selections either.

It might have been expected that all three were obvious in deciding to play, but the obvious isn't so obvious when it comes to Age-defying Athletes.

Algorithms need not apply

At the launch of this project, the assumption was that mature adults would have taken an analytical approach to sport selection.

Online are dozens of "sport match" sites which encourage the user to answer questions such as "Do you like to challenge yourself?" and "Do you like to be outdoors?" Results are scrubbed by an algorithm, and *voila!*, out pops the best sport fit.

But only 12% of ADAP respondents reported having reviewed more than one sport, and these reviews were primarily informal. No one took the algorithmic pathway to athletic happiness.

Lack of childhood sports involvement

A hefty portion of the ADAP sample – 41% - never swatted a bat or kicked a ball as children. Perhaps there was the occasional backyard badminton game at a birthday party, or the mandatory physical education (PE) class which many managed to evade anyway.

Nor did they ever expect that as adults they would become pickleball players, swimmers, golfers, bikers, tennis enthusiasts, squash players, marathoners, softball team members, rowers, ping-pong players, yogis, or triathletes.

As with seeds that unexpectedly blossom in the garden, however, there was a mysterious mix of elements – maybe time, people, situation, dreams? - and the next thing you know, shazam! A bunch of unexpected, Age-defying Athletes, declared, "Hello, World!"

Here are a two of those with no sports background who sipped the brew and were revitalized.

Georgette

Georgette, 61, is a good example of an Age-defying Athlete who came to the game of golf with no childhood sporting experiences - other than cheerleading.

"I am left-handed, shy, and had no nerve to ask people how to teach a sport to someone left-handed."

Her husband wanted her to learn golf, but it took her ten years to finally agree. Not only that, but at first, she was "too embarrassed to play with anyone besides my husband and two friends."

Eventually, Georgette drank deeply of the sport nectar. But she was still stymied by her skill. "I discovered that I want to fit in, but when I was so bad, I didn't fit in! I had to get over it...I wish I'd started sooner."

Georgette began playing about six years ago and has achieved a 25 handicap. She golfs four times a week.

The key benefit of playing golf, she maintains, is that she has "more friends than I've ever had."

Isaac

"I went to school and then I went to work," he reports. "Beginning at age 13, I was picking cotton in the summertime. The next summer, when I was 14, I could drive to the fields to pick. Both years, we camped there and picked cotton."

Isaac, 86, continues: "I worked through college, so no sports. College was night school because I worked for a railroad during the day, later working days for an oil company. I was a musician on the side, starting in 1957, playing Friday and Saturday nights."

As was the case with some other ADAP respondents, Isaac's job nudged him toward the game. He began at the urging of guys in the office.

"...1960, age 25. My colleagues told me to buy a tennis racquet and to come out and play with them. That's how I learned. We played Thursday nights, then later more nights. Mostly singles.

"But I never had occasion to commit to a group. I'd play with one group for a few months, and then for various reasons, I'd move to a new group."

Unfolding his story, Isaac adds, "The last ten years I worked, I traveled a lot, and was just on a sub list. Played erratically. I retired at age 57 with the hope to get back to the game and improve."

In 1994, retirement brought him to Orange Beach, Alabama.

"I started playing singles and doubles six days a week. I saw an ad for tennis lessons plus a playing group in Gulf

Shores and signed up. There I met people who told me about another place, so I signed up for that, too. Over there, I learned about another center. I became friends with people all around the Gulf coast."

He still plays three times weekly, and says of the game, "Wonderful experience throughout my life."

Ample childhood sports involvement

At the other extreme from zero sports background are those who had a ton of it.

The vast majority of interviewees in ADAP - 79% - did not picture themselves as future athletes.

However, of those 21% who did, a couple were on Olympic Games tracks, and had some rationale for this expectation.

As Natalya's story, below, illustrates, however, youthful athletic achievement does not necessarily pave a smooth path to adult sports selections.

Natalya

One of these former athletic *wunderkinds* is 55-year-old Natalya who lives in the southern US.

"I did [expect to become an athlete]. My brothers and I would stand on three large rocks in our backyard, pretending to accept Olympic medals. They were in soccer and track."

Unfortunately, childhood aspiration is always subject to the vagaries of chance, as Natalya discovered.

"I was a competitive swimmer from age five through high school. I loved swimming, actually was on an AAU track to the Olympics when I missed the trials by 1/100th of a second. One bad day and my career crashed."

Despite this disappointment, Natalya stuck with sports. While still in high school, she moved over to cross-country and track.

She continued to run for another 15 years, then had an epiphany. "After high school, I ran 5K, 10K until [my] mid-thirties, then realized I didn't like running."

Following that, she played no sports, just swam and worked out. (Swimming is in her blood, however, as she continues that sport to this very day.)

Sports are all about functional fitness. That is, muscles that are trained are the muscles that grow strong; the moves that are practiced are the moves that become instinctive.

Despite her impressive history of athletic accomplishment, Natalya had never played ball sports. "I had no hand-eye coordination." This would come back to haunt her when she started playing golf.

In the early 21st century, scientists from the University of Chicago found that there are neurological differences between how a beginner and an advanced player approach the game. They identified three differences:[16]

"First, skills are voluntary goal-directed sequences of movements.

"Second, practice is required to both attain and to maintain the skill level.

"<u>Third, skills exhibit specificity, i.e., the skill level is not directly transferable to other skills.</u>" (Emphasis added.)

Ironically, the more advanced an athlete becomes in any given sport, the more difficult it can be to translate that sport's skills to a different type of game.

Natalya's outstanding athletic background would not easily migrate to the new game of golf (hand-eye coordination, remember?), which Natalya decided to try about two-and-a-half years ago.

"My husband had been playing four or five years. He took lessons in a nearby town. By then I had stopped teaching [history in high school] and my husband wanted me to play, but I kept saying 'no'."

In fact, it took her almost twelve months to decide to take the plunge: "The most difficult aspect of starting was just knowing that I had to make a four-and-a-half hour [time] commitment."

Confounding her reluctance, she explains, "I didn't know what club to use, how to score, nuances, distances. All this took awhile to master."

Finally, it dawned on her "that I would have to try because I didn't want to be a golf widow. So, I started playing and took some lessons, and then it clicked and I loved it."

Quite a number of ADAP participants have discovered things about themselves by playing a sport. Natalya did, too.

"I discovered that my patience is not what I thought, and I am hard on myself. I wasn't competitive with other people, but with myself."

Another discovery – this one a surprise - was "that I could do it and that I would like it... Plus, I am thankful to see older women healthy and playing, they are role models, and I hope to continue golfing into my 70s. It's been fun."

No kidding

By her decision to golf, Natalya ultimately made a surprise discovery: she found this competent, happy person having fun, and that person was she. That's self-renewing.

Isaac's decision led him to a wonderful lifelong experience. How different would his life have been if he hadn't elected to try tennis? That's self-renewing.

Georgette, Hans, Belinda, Langley, Felicity, Veronica, Borden, Sam, Winston, Cora, Reynaldo, and the others - even imaginary Dagny - have all tasted the elixir of sport and have been rejuvenated.

And there's no kidding about that.

Chapter 4
Preparing to play

To lesson or not to lesson?

"I took Saturday drills, lessons. I am a rules-based person and if I understand how the rules work, I am better. Practice makes permanent."

Vs.

"I have a problem with lessons. The golf swing has the same components, so I should be able to go to different pros and have them tell me the same thing. But this isn't so. Each pro has his or her own idea of what I should be doing. They want to change my golf swing, and that makes my score drop. Each pro will change your game. I prefer to read the fundamentals and do it myself."

These quotes summarize the two poles that Age-defying Athletes faced after an elixir sip inspired them to jump off the cliff of their predictable lives and hurl themselves into sport space.

These poles represent the two basic approaches toward athletic preparation: Take lessons or do-it-yourself?

Lessons being a third person phenomenon: someone else provides feedback. This feedback could come during a one-to-one lesson, clinic, drill, camp, rookie (or supervised learn-by-playing) league, "buddy" program, or multi-day intensive.

Do-it-yourself (DIY) being a first person phenomenon: the player trusts his or her senses to figure out how a game is played. They may do a lot of real-time observation, read books, watch videos and TV, and/or simply go out and try it.

76% of the Age-defying Athletes profiled in this book took lessons, while the other 24% were DIYers.

Stats wobble

As crisp as those statistics may appear in this decidedly unscientific study, they contain a couple of wobblies.

One wobbly is that a few in the lesson camp initially went out a time or two (or more) on their own to pursue the game in question. But they quickly realized that they needed formal third-party guidance.

This, for instance, was the case with the only pickleball player who took lessons. She did that after having tried the game for a while.

Another wobbly is that anything that provides third party feedback falls into "lesson". Age-defying Athletes tended not to discriminate amongst all those lesson models. So, those methods are all represented in the "lessons" stat.

Further, some of the "instructors" were actually spouses. Fascinating to contemplate the feedback dynamic of that...

How Athletes sorted themselves regarding preparation

Golfers were more consistently students of someone else, while tennis players tended to inhabit the DIY ranks.

One triathlete was involved in intensive group trainings for months, whereas another "tri" couple simply read a book and started competing.

Reynaldo (Chapter 3), a sportsman solidly in the DIY column also read a book to develop his marathon training regimen.

Interestingly, these two bookish ones both have PhDs.

In contrast (oh those ornery Doctors of Philosophy), two other PhDs read no books, but just went out and bicycled and swam.

In contrast to this contrast, Veronica (Chapter 3), another PhD, not only took lessons as a rookie rower, but continues to take coaching today.

Running, bicycling and swimming are individual sports, and no individual sport athlete in ADAP (except for the female triathlete) took lessons. Maybe that's part of the appeal of these solo sports? The rugged individualism of DIY?

Lesson pros and cons

Even among those who used lessons to prepare to play, there was disagreement about their efficacy.

Gigi

One beginner who thrived with lessons is Gigi.

"She's always coming up with new ideas," noted the affable gentleman who is Gigi's husband. "Travel, entertaining, rehabbing this place, that vegetable garden..."

Gigi responds, "It's a personality trait that I try to figure out how to do something well."

She had focused on career and family for 30 years, so why take up tennis at age 51?

"I just up and did it. I usually jump into things. Not afraid of looking bad...Took early retirement, then was busy [in a second career]. Needed exercise. On a lark, decided to learn tennis."

This zesty 73-year-old describes how she prepared for this new game:

"I bought a Target® tennis racquet, can of balls, and a cute black visor with pink stripes."

Gigi relates what happened next, "Our local club advertised a drop-in lesson held over three consecutive days. I went to it and discovered that it was for more advanced players. I couldn't hit the ball. The pro felt bad.

"So I took more lessons to learn how to hit the ball. These were at 7AM once a week, and I went to work afterward."

"Staying with it," she explains, "was the hard part. Tennis requires incredible focus, and I have to really work at watching the ball.

"But I'm a natural student, so I liked the lessons and have never stopped taking them."

Ramona

Gigi relishes lessons. But Ramona is more neutral about them, stating, "I could give a lesson on golf lessons."

Here's what happened to this 77-year-old golfer.

"In one facility, I used an old [golf club] set of my husband's. I took six lessons and was only taught to use the nine iron, so I wondered what am I supposed to do with the other clubs?"

Ramona continues, "I had a horrendous job, worked long hours, so for classes, I would often get there late, and the pro would be angry. I just didn't have the time."

Changing the lesson circumstances, unfortunately, produced unchanging results. "Another club pro," she reports, "commented once, 'I'm sure you're surprised that someone like yourself can hit a golf ball.' It was a surprising comment, that's for sure."

DIY pros and cons

The do-it-yourself segment also had true believers and lukewarm acolytes.

Hazel

Frequently, the DIY enthusiast is motivated by a sense of urgency. Hazel is a good example.

"My husband and I were in bed on a Saturday morning,"

states Hazel, 74, "And I said I had something to tell him: I want to play golf. He replied that he was happy he was still in bed, because otherwise he would have fallen over.

"I told him that if we don't do something together, we'll kill each other or divorce. He wanted to wait and borrow equipment, but I said, no, we are going to the store today and making a financial commitment – we bought clubs, clothes, etc. We could afford the sport and I now had time. All in."

Lukewarm acolytes of the DIY faith learn (ha) that that in the long run it can be far less efficient and much slower to go out and "do it" than to confer with a pro. Norbert provides an object lesson about this.

Norbert

"Nothing really," responds Norbert, 77, when asked how he prepared for tennis. "I have never taken a lesson or attended a clinic. Learned by doing."

His espousal of the DIY creed is tempered by the fact that he has had a hit-or-miss experience.

"However, when I came back [to tennis at age 62, two decades since he participated as a young man], I expected it would only take a few months until I achieved the level of play I enjoyed when I stopped at age 42. But it took five to seven years to reach my 20 years' younger level."

Deciding to lesson or not

With these pros and cons of lessons and DIY, what tips a given athlete toward one preparation philosophy or another?

Goals

One factor is the objective of playing in the first place. If the goal is to meet people when relocating to a new community, just going out and playing may suffice.

But if the sportsperson is interested in bringing home a trophy or making the family proud, more formal instruction may be needed.

Sport starting point

Another factor influencing prep selection is sport starting point: Sports Virgin? Prodigal? Continuer?

Sports Virgins – people who have inconsequential or no history with their sport of choice. These rookies aren't simply stepping beyond their comfort zones in pursuit of golf glory or tennis thrills – they are bounding into the unknown. On the other hand, their expectations tend to be low, and their bodies are in the present – unlike the "past" (or remembered) bodies inhabited by Prodigals and Continuers.

Prodigals - men and women who are hitting the "on" switch after years of being "off". Unlike beginners, they have a sense about what to expect from a game. But their bodies and minds are older than they were in their prime playing years. Despite this, given that the games are still perceived by them to be within their comfort zones, Prodigals likely anticipate starting right back up, playing as they did ten, twenty, or more years ago.

Continuers - these people decide...well, continually...to go out and play. Since they never really stopped throwing or hopping or catching, their comfort zones have grown large enough to accommodate their level and style of play. Unlike for rookies, Continuers have little or no novelty with which to grapple. But as with Prodigals, Continuers' performance expectations are high and perhaps outdated. Wear and tear on the corpus mechanism are keenly felt.

Here are a few ADAP examples of how the sport starting point influenced the choice of preparation modality.

Sports virgins prepare to play

Not surprisingly, across all the team sports, Sports Virgins or rookies tended to take lessons – sometimes many, sometimes just one or two.

Jacinta

Jacinta, a 75-year-old golfer who first stepped onto the links five years ago, describes how she started: "I took a lot of lessons with a pro. Also took [indoor] lessons and practiced [at the indoor facility], especially when weather was bad. We would go there three or four times a week."

She continues: "We took couples introductory course offered by our club and that made a difference. The pro instructor was very straightforward and tells it like it is. That works for me."

On the other hand, some beginners took no lessons. They may have recognized they had no skill in a particular game, but were more confident about the ease of picking up the sport. After all, they had learned to play many games in their lifetimes, so how hard could this be?

Crawford

Crawford is a 66-year-old tennis player who jumped into the game at the urging of her sister-in-law about eight years ago. "I never took lessons. Just went out and played."

A perfectionist, Crawford adds, "For me, when I do something, don't like not to do it well. So I had to become skilled enough [on my own at tennis] that I didn't think that way. Tennis is more forgiving than golf."

Prodigals plan a return

What's the best way to step back into a game after a decade or more absence? There is no "best" way, of course, but the ramp-up probably reflects a timeline (Play next week or play after an event next year?) and a recollection of past skill.

Nate

Following a decade-long hiatus from tennis, Nate cycled back to the game and started taking lessons. "When I was 40," reports this 73-year-old who plays tennis three times a week, "I took clinics and some private lessons. I still do [take a weekly lesson]. Absolutely learn by watching."

Carmella

Another accomplished tennis player returned on the DIY bus. "Using my old racquet – a very old racquet," recalls Carmella who came back to tennis after 15 years away from the game, "I went to the [city] courts and hit against the backboard there. Then, I bought a new racquet and joined [our club's] fun tennis."

Continuers may need recalibration – or not

Did Continuers grudgingly admit that a tune-up here and there was needed?

Some did, some didn't.

Victoria

Victoria, 71, falls into the first category. She has played tennis for almost 50 years and notes that today her goal is

"Keep on playing. It always feels good to win, but I am not upset if I lose."

She still utilizes third-person instruction. "Used to take a lot of lessons. More clinics now, due to their better affordability."

Tyrel

In contrast, a five decades and counting tennis Continuer is Tyrel, 76. He states, "When we moved to [our current town], my game needed sprucing up. [My wife] took lots of lessons, but I have only taken two my entire life. So, I learned by failing along the way."

Will it be hard to learn?

Another factor influencing preparation selection is perception of how arduous the task promises to be. That is, if the task or sport is thought to be complex (like the game of squash, say), then the athlete may tend more toward outside help.

But for something viewed as straightforward and accessible, like riding a bike (so accessible, in fact, "you never forget how to ride a bike" has slipped into our vernacular to represent an action to be quickly picked up), DIY is okey dokey.

But, of course, what's accessible to a Continuer may be perceived as impossible to a Virgin.

For the former, high attained skill needs to be balanced by a high level of challenge in order for play to be fulfilling.

For the latter, attained skill can only handle a low level of challenge.

Each player must find some sort of equilibrium between ability and perceived task challenge. And equilibrium will possibly oscillate over time.

The tradeoff between ability and challenge is captured by a concept called "Flow".

Flow is not a training technique, *per se*. In the context of lessons/DIY, Flow serves as a gauge of athlete skill building.

For example, following many months of training (DIY or third party) and play, the new golfer still racks up nine-hole scores in the 60s. Looks like the task challenge is higher than the skill level. But then, sometime later, after more instruction, golfer scores begin to float into the 50s for nine. Skill is catching up with challenge. The conclusion is that the preparation approach is effective – finally.

On the other hand, if the new golfer - after just a couple of lessons - shoots in the 50s almost from the start, task is below skill. Perhaps a different course may offer more of an equal challenge to ability.

Flow

This tradeoff between ability and challenge is the idea of "flow"[17] promulgated by the psychologist Mihaly Csikszentmihalyi. Flow is an equilibrium point: too much challenge for a given skill level causes anxiety; too much skill for a particular challenge induces boredom.

In other words, people want to achieve without falling asleep or being scared to death.

In sports, the "Flow" athlete is so involved with the experience, he or she doesn't monitor the skill or the challenge – it's all about the rhythm of doing. Athletes are effortlessly flowing through the movement...at one with it.

Csikszentmihalyi's "Flow" might be likened to being "in the zone".

Reaching the zone is an objective of preparation (lessons or DIY), as it matches the perceived difficulty of mastering a sport with the learned skill.

Not to mention that being in the zone also contributes to the sense of renewal experienced by athletes.

ADAPers in the zone – or not
Lawton

A golfer who began playing golf over 40 years ago, Lawton, 77, expresses his zone as "From time to time, rewarding to get better, to hit a straight drive or drop a 30 foot putt. Temporary euphoria."

Euphoria, for sure, but also reinforcement that Lawton has – at least occasionally – found that balance between the skill he needs for golf and the challenge of the links.

Gundun

At 79, Gundun has played tennis for decades, and finds her type of "Flow" in interacting with others. "Keeps me younger to be around younger people."

She elaborates that "Tennis is best way to take your mind off whatever bothers you and just focus on the game. Feel better every time I walk off court. Any time I exercise, I feel better."

Juanita – not flowing

Disequilibrium, on the other hand, imperils Flow and renewal, as this ADAP respondent can attest.

Juanita, 64, is a retired executive who has worked all over the world and achieved career success. She is also a polysport (playing both golf and tennis) who started on the links almost 35 years ago.

Now retired, Juanita is a very capable golfer. But she finds herself at an imbalance – not so much between skill and challenge, but, instead, between the desire to have fun and the need to be challenged. Basically, she seeks the state of Flow in golf but finds that it escapes her.

"I try to have fun. I would like to get to a place where I don't care [about my golf performance]," laments Juanita.

"People who can laugh at themselves have more fun, even if they aren't as good. But what is the point of not being good?," she wonders.

"Can't have ups and downs. When I tried not to care about ups and downs, I didn't have fun because I couldn't remember my good shots."

Juanita claims that "Tennis is more consistent. I can play tennis and shut down my brain without ruining my game."

A similar disequilibrium is expressed by under-50 tennis player, Nelli, in Chapter 9.

Flow is for all athlete levels

Mike Csikszentmihalyi might not have agreed with this, but Flow needn't be limited to expert players. Just as long as skill level and challenge are matched, a player can achieve the state, enhancing ability and boosting confidence.

For example, the beginning tennis player may find fluid rhythm merely hitting a ball against a backboard. No tremendous skill is required, and the challenge is predictable and circumscribed.

Similarly, the new golfer can enter a zone by hitting balls at the driving range. In fact, a subset of golfers prefers the range to the course for this very reason.

Reaching the zone is possible for a player at any level. Certainly, this can be a benefit to beginners. It reinforces learning and builds confidence.

THE ELIXIR OF SPORT

Being a rookie isn't all bad

Since lots of readers of this book may be Sports Virgins, it's good to recognize that newbies enjoy special benefits more advanced people don't.

As Tom Vanderbilt points out in his book, *Beginners*,[18] greenhorns have the advantage of low expectations. With low hurdles, it is okay to be rough around the edges, untutored.

During learning, the rookie brain is sucking in a lot of novelty and awareness…and mistakes. But mistakes train the brain about the novel undertaking. Rather than beating up on themselves about a topped golf ball or a tennis double fault, players would do well to learn from the moment and move on.

There is a state, in fact, called the "perpetual novice" – those who continue to master new things while making mistakes and learning from them along the way.[19]

Ironically, as the novice (perpetual or otherwise) becomes more advanced, he or she faces a burden. Because as one climbs the expertise ladder, possible solutions to problems ("Why does my backhand always go wide?") are crowded out by the "purity" of one's supposed expertise ("I can't believe I did that; I haven't hit wide since last year.").

Another thing Vanderbilt reports is that beginner-beginner friendships are more easily formed than expert-expert friendships, in which status and competitiveness tend to muck up the works.

Despite all these advantages, Sports Virgins understandably want to move on to higher and higher levels of proficiency. How does skill advancement occur?

Five Stages of Learning

Turns out, an informative five stage model of skill acquisition was proposed by Hubert Dreyfus and Stuart Dreyfus in their book *Mind over Machine*.[20]

The basic idea is that a novice proceeds from a rules-based initial approach through four further phases until the skill becomes intuitive, Flowing, "in the zone".

The five stages are:

1. Novice: Learn facts, figures, rules without any context or situation, e.g., the pickleball serve
2. Advanced Beginner: Learn how to apply rules in various situations, e.g., the pickleball serve targeting a particular spot in the receiver box
3. Competent: Learn how to prioritize rules and techniques as the situation changes, e.g., pickleball serve to lefty when the score is 10-9-2 vs. when the score is 10-9-1
4. Proficient: Incorporate intuition into the playing of pickleball so that it's more about a "feel" for the game, e.g., pickleball serve to lefty at 10-9-2 predicting what the competitor will expect and doing something different
5. Expert: Just moving through the game intuitively, without thinking about serving (or anything else) in any particular way

Since all athletes are Novices at one point or another, it is informative to look further at the beginning stage of skill acquisition.

Q: What really distinguishes the Novice from the Advanced Beginner?

A: A stuffed brain

Or, as Tom Vanderbilt puts it more elegantly, "For the novice, everything is important, and everything warrants his or her attention."[21]

For example, the newbie golfer thinks hard about where her wrists, elbows, hips, and head are in the backswing and agonizes about her rotation. Once she reaches expertise, she is one with the club and simply swings.

Learning, in effect, is a process of discarding anything that is not critical to the task at hand. Or, put differently, learning shifts from "How to-s" to "Do-s", from rules to intuition. The athlete becomes the game.

The neuroscience insight

This concept of the overloaded greenhorn brain vs. the uncluttered expert brain has a neurological grounding, as shown in research work conducted on professional and amateur female golfers by the University of Chicago in the early years of this century.

In a paper entitled *On the Road to Automatic: Dynamic Aspects in the Development of Expertise*,[22] the scientists explore what distinguishes expert motor skills from more undeveloped skills.

The authors write:

"One of the important steps on the road to becoming expert in a motor skill occurs when the individual can perform the movements in a seemingly effortless and automatic fashion."[23] (Emphasis added.)

This is what Dreyfus would term the fifth or Expert Stage of Learning.

The University of Chicago scientists continue:

"...this road to automatic involves two steps: (1) an increasing reliance on the self-regulatory aspects of the motor task, and (2) a minimization of the role of mechanisms based on intentionally directed corrective movements. The interplay between these two mechanisms implies that, at a given skill level, performance decreases whenever intention intervenes. (Emphasis added.)

"The observation that psychological factors may be as important as mechanical repetition for the development of expertise has important implications for the design of neurorehabilitative strategies."[24]

What is thought of as skill development is basically starting down that road toward automatic, progressing toward the intuitive expert level in the Five Stages of Learning.

In the beginning, sportsters have to think about moving arms, legs, and body, but need to stop thinking about these things as they improve. Improvement, in fact, should be viewed as thinking less and less.

With respect to preparation, when traveling down the road to automatic, the athlete could be steering the wheel themselves.

Or, they could invite a third-party to do the driving via lessons, clinics, drills, camps.

Learning style also influences choice of prep

For both self-steerers and those in the "passenger seat," learning style can influence the choice of preparation mode.

Visual learners learn best when they can see something – a move, written instructions, symbols.

Betje

Betje, 64, decided to learn golf after a lifetime of "disastrous" golfing vacations with her family.

"I decided I would get serious or quit," she says. "I worked with the [indoor technology facility] coach and I did all the lessons. Practice time. Every other week. I decided to try it because someone recommended it. Club pro was good, but I needed something more and [facility] records each swing. I am a visual learner."

Mirroring

Mirroring can be thought of as another educational style related to visual learning. Like visual-only teaching techniques, it can be utilized in lessons or when doing-it-yourself.

As the name implies, the learner watches a movement – Tiger Woods hitting a pitching wedge or Venus Williams covering the net, for example – and then tries to replicate it. Visual input can come from a real person (perhaps a pro demonstrating a move), a video, a TV match, even from a photo or picture. In this way, it blends visual and kinesthetic styles.

The idea behind mirroring is that specific neurons fire both when an activity is observed as well as when it is performed. This repetition strengthens the neural pathway, which enhances cognition (and skill).

Mildred

Mirroring was useful for Mildred, a 73-year-old tennis player who returned to the game after treatment for cancer.

"Breast cancer was diagnosed in May 2020 and I had to back off [tennis] about six months. I would hit a bit, but couldn't play a serious game."

Her biggest challenge "...coming back was mobility and strength in my left arm." Previously a two-handed backhand hitter, Mildred "worked with drills to learn one-handed backhand again."

"When developing this one-hand stroke, I thought of Steffi Graf's one-handed backhand."

A bonus of this experience was that "In the process of developing a new backhand, I learned to slice, which I had never had."

Auditory learners learn best from sound - listening to an explanation or a description.

Brett

When he became serious about golf, Brett, 68, first sought to listen to an experienced linksman. "As time became less and less of a problem, I went to range and took advice from a good golfer."

He then augmented this with formal training: "First lesson probably age 56, which was four days of golf school in the desert."

He says that bad habits are hard to change, but the desert school utilized sensors to record various aspects of the swing. This helped him develop an appreciation of the technical aspects of the game.

As Brett's story demonstrates, mixing learning style techniques can be effective.

Gail

Another golfer, Gail, 66, relied on conversations. "I started with a Pro and [then] joined LGA. They have Big Sis & Little Sis program - mentors for beginners."

Kinesthetic learners need to feel the move – the rhythm of weight transfer, the pull of water as an arm is lifted for a swimming stroke. Kinesthetic types tend to be "just do it" learners.

Francisco

Francisco, 79, is a good example of a DIY learner who is kinesthetic.

"I find enjoyment in being outdoors and improving at something difficult. Sheer joy of smacking golf ball on screws on a pretty day with your buddies."

Preparation evolves.

What's more, athletes ignore preparation direction at their peril.

Just as athletes evolve from beginners to experts, preparation should evolve, too.

Tennis-playing Gigi offers insights on this transition:

"Different pros are needed at different phases of tennis development. Beginners need a pro who can teach the fundamentals, all the shots.

"Once the player is more advanced, he or she needs a pro who can work on court movement, where to be, and when.

"Beyond that, you need a pro who can work with your head, and teach you how to put together a point. And, of course, any pro must be compatible with your personality."

And it goes without saying – though it will be stated here anyway – the player must incorporate the preparation into his or her performance. This applies whether or not the sportsperson took third-party lessons or is self-taught.

Eventually – but not at first – Age-defying Athletes Winston and Cora followed both precepts after a fashion.

Winston and Cora

Their New Hampshire house was silent. Winston and his wife Cora rolled around in it like marbles.

It had seemed only yesterday that the place reverberated with laughter from three little kids – five, six, and seven.

As the years had progressed, there was the parade of kid teams – soccer, baseball, football – with plenty of noise about battles lost, battles won, and the clatter of equipment in all the places it shouldn't be.

Teenage dramas, wrestling with authority, seeking advice, music, clothes, college, careers, people clanged and crashed from room to room.

Now, just a hushed house filled with two empty-nesters...

Winston, 71, earned a doctorate and had a career in geology. Cora (a few years younger) was in a literary field.

Growing up on the east coast, this PhD had been in just about every sport available.

"I was pushed into six years of baseball; that was [my] main sport as a kid," he declares. "But I played a lot of pick-up games, stick ball, a lot more neighborhood play that was unorganized, almost continuous.

"In high school, I did cross country and track."

Cross country and track were rewarding, but also frustrating. "I got tendonitis on top of my foot and it was painful," he reports. "If we had had modern shoes, it wouldn't happen, but back then, running shoes were heavy leather with no cushioning".

The inflammation happened at a meet. "The coach at the track event put a rolled-up ball of gauze behind my toes and the pain immediately went away," recalls Winston. He competed successfully.

"However, the next day, I couldn't walk. Thankfully, sports medicine had advanced since then."

Winston continued with cross-country throughout college. But then stopped in grad school.

Instead, when he went to the University of New Hampshire, he took up cross-country skiing "...and have cross country skied for the rest of my life."

Throughout it all, the common thread was cardio and endurance sports, which grew from his cross-country experiences. Ironically, he practiced these irregularly.

"I would periodically have 'fitness' bouts," Winston admits " – kind of parallel to lapsed Catholics - in which my fits of remorse at having sinned for growing flabby and unfit brought me back to running on and off."

Winston avers that when he was growing up, the high school and college mindset was that if you "do cardio", you don't "do strength" (i.e., play football), so "...there was a certain disrespect for strength training which was not a good thing."

By the 1970s, Winston was into a wide range of distance running training, following a smorgasbord of regimens.

He recalls that "When I returned for triathlons, all these myriad regimens had coalesced into a single regimen called periodicity. Slow, then fast workouts based on calendars."

Significantly, due to his youthful loyalty to the church of separation of cardio and strength, he needed to ...well... strengthen strength. "When tri started, you had to do strength."

In contrast to Winston's extensive game-playing resume as a youth, Cora was never in competitive sports.

They weren't the most likely couple to start participating in triathlons.

Nonetheless, "My wife and I fell into it," Winston explains about their decision. "We were becoming empty nesters and she bought a book, *Slow Fat Triathlete*."[25]

It appealed to this retired geologist right away. "The road running part hearkened back to my cross country days."

He continues, "There are four triathlon levels, mostly reflecting distance for each of the three sports (swim, bike, run): sprint is shortest, then Olympic, half Ironman, and Ironman.

"Our goal became to finish a sprint triathlon, so we jumped into a six-week program."

"There was no formal instruction, just self-coached," he reminisces. "But for awhile, we joined our local facility's triathlon club, and that was helpful for bicycling and open water swimming. Their Masters Swim program was also very beneficial.

"The first [event] was in Bar Harbor, Maine, a gorgeous setting. We drank a lot of wine the night before, and the event was a total disaster for us. We did all the wrong things."

"Naturally," Winston warms to the tale, "we decided, 'That was so bad, we have to do it again.' And then we were off. This became an excuse to travel and we got the bug."

Once they realized that they needed to be more serious about the sport, they followed a periodicity plan.

"[The plan] called for building one's base of endurance during the off season," Winston elucidates. "Once the season rolled around, we moved to high intensity training. We used to sprint on bicycles up the [local mountain] road for two to three minutes, then coast downhill...and we did that a lot."

The couple got into it in a big way, with heart monitors, training zones, aerobic to anaerobic protocols. "We discovered that staying aerobic led to better performance in the long run."

Winston became a periodicity fan: "Periodicity really works, keeps burnout at bay, because it forces regular rest. With periodicity, there are three light months annually."

Triathlon competition, the couple discovered, wasn't always great. They had to learn to eat while in the act. Winston threw up the first time on those gummy "meals".

Gummy meals or no, for the next six years, Winston and Cora participated in five to six events annually.

During that time, as might be expected of a brainy couple, "We often talked about 'Where are we going with this?' But the 'tri' aspect is good because if you are sick of running, for instance, you can just focus on single sporting events in swimming and bicycling for awhile."

On the other hand, the old saying is that "tri people" can no longer compete in single events, argues Winston, "...so they rely on the three sport model to boost their chances: You can't win on the swim, but you can lose. People usually win on their run performance, rarely on swimming. But it's always possible.

"One other thing is that it's easier for older people to try new things because they are less concerned about looking foolish than younger people."

Cora had trouble with knees and hips, so her running was hampered. But the cross training helped minimize injury.

And, he proudly proclaims, "My wife, for her age group, was outstanding due to my coaching (!not!)."

When he took a new job across the USA, they had to cut back.

Triathlon participation delivered an "enormous fitness benefit. Introducing biking and swimming to my running history was a great benefit. I really love swimming and find it almost meditative."

He concludes that the sport delivers "Fitness and general well being, even mental."

Winston then adds, however, "I don't miss awakening at 6 am to go out and stand on a dark beach waiting for the triathlon to begin."

Preparation: another step on the road to renewal

Whether or not Age-defying Athletes took lessons, did it themselves, or some combination of these, they sought something novel...something that would change them.

It doesn't matter whether or not they knew what this changed self would look like. It was just important that they prepared to step out of their past and into their future.

Chapter 5
Playing

*What happens when adults sip
the playing elixir?*

What happens is that Age-defying Athletes evolve into new versions of themselves – or, rather, they liberate something new, fresh, and "young" that had been inside them all along.

Having moved through two life-cycle stages – the decision to try something new, the preparation (in their own ways) for this new thing - Age-defying Athletes now are out there, drinking the brew, and performing the new.

Of course, the "new" is not a single experience. Rather, it's like 92 different experiences, because each Age-defying Athlete perceives the whole magilla differently than all the others.

What happens when they play?

Plenty of things happen, of course, but the focus in this Chapter is on the level of satisfaction enjoyed (or not) by members of the ADAP community.

The top line is that ADAP interviewees can be arrayed along a spectrum stretching from sort of OK on the left, to somewhat positive in the middle, with very positive on the right – or low to high satisfaction from left to right.

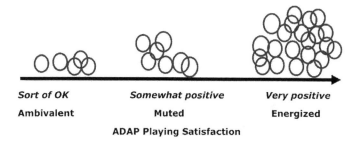

Sort of OK   **Somewhat positive**   **Very positive**
Ambivalent   Muted   Energized

ADAP Playing Satisfaction

These satisfaction zones are defined as Ambivalent, Muted, and Energized.

The largest clump of respondents are on the right or Energized end; moving left are fewer "somewhat positives" (Muted) and continuing leftward, even thinner ranks occupying "sort of OK" (Ambivalent).

This satisfaction spectrum will be brought to life by Athletes' own stories.

Sport characteristics

But first, what are some sport characteristics that may cause an Athlete to land in a given spot on the spectrum?

Five key ones will be discussed here: frequency, format, skill, consistency, and competition. Comments about short-term factors will be included, but their overall impact is difficult to gauge.

Frequency and format are straightforward reports on what occurs. As such, they may provide limited insights about Age-defying Athletes' satisfaction or dissatisfaction.

The more frequently someone plays a game, for instance, the more likely they are (a) to like it and (b) to get better at it. (The question being, of course, which comes first, the liking or the improvement?)

As far as format is concerned, it's probably safe to say that introverts tend toward solo sports and extroverts, toward those built on groups. If players are properly aligned, this will lead to greater satisfaction, all other things being equal.

The latter three characteristics – skill, consistency, and competition - will provide a richer idea of what drives ADAP respondents to be very positive, somewhat positive, or sort of OK about their playing.

Deeper dives into each sport characteristic contributing to satisfaction

Frequency

Participating, they definitely are! After all their deliberations and get-ready-to-play, these Athletes want to have at it.

The 34 tennis players go out and play, on average, three times a week, with a couple of the most fervent competing almost daily. They primarily play doubles tennis.

Golfers – totaling 39 in ADAP – also average three rounds a week, with heaviest hitters taking to the links four times every seven days.

Pickleball players total eight in number and they play about two times a week, with a range of one to four outings.

The softball player participates in two or three games a week during the season.

The swimmer jumps into the pool three times a week.

Triathletes and marathoners generally compete a couple of times a year.

The squash player goes out about twice weekly.

So, too, do the two bicyclists.

Ping-pong has been occasional, but is soon going to happen more regularly.

The rower is "on the water" four times weekly.

And the yoga adherent practices once or twice a month – with the hope that this will happen more often in the future.

How frequency influences satisfaction

For one thing, frequency numbers indicate that Age-defying Athletes return again and again to their sports. Irrespective of where they fall on the satisfaction spectrum, they are committed. And this commitment is a key building block of the renewal they enjoy.

Additionally, these statistics suggest that the players have a pretty good idea of what sports participation entails, irrespective of whether or not they are Sports Virgins, Prodigals, or Continuers. They are living what they preach, even if they are still struggling with beginner-itis.

In terms of where they land on the "love it" to "meh" satisfaction spectrum, high frequency sportspeople may tend to be more comfortable with a sport and participate more because they get a lot from it – again irrespective of their playing skill. Conversely, those who just come out sporadically may not be as committed to a game and feel more "on the fence" about it.

Format

Solo sports

First, the solitary ones. Bicycle and swim enthusiasts are solo athletes, electing non-competitive versions of their sports. They do not participate on Masters' Swim teams or race with herds of MAMIS (Middle-Aged Men In Spandex).

Rowing can be done in a one-person boat, or in an eight-rower scull.

Reynaldo, the marathoner, runs against everyone in the race, so his is a solo pursuit but with competition. In like fashion are Winston and Cora, the triathlete couple, and Ling, a triathlete woman.

Golf is a trickier format to characterize. A single golfer can certainly revel in a round, and many feel that golf is a solitary pursuit.

But most of the individuals in ADAP hit the course with others. "Others" include spouses, family members, or friends.

Also, "others" may be league participants in which a duffer partners with another player(s) and vies against other two- or foursomes.

These leagues frequently extend beyond one particular course, supporting a network of "traveling" teams.

Samantha, a golf pro in Texas, explains interclub play among eleven clubs: "Each [club] fields a team of eight. [There are] eleven play days [throughout the year] but the date your club hosts the event your team doesn't play and runs the tournament. Works out great. We host the opening event in March. We have 15 women on our team and our captains make sure we each get at least two events to play."

Like golf, yoga is an individual endeavor usually practiced within a group. As Ingrid, a 59-year-old yogini explains, "You do your own class on the mat, but [experience] a lot of camaraderie before, during, and after."

Group sports

It's tough to play racquet sports by oneself (!), so ADAP racquet-wielders engage in recreational or organized group competition.

Recreational tennis/pickleball/squash/ping-pong may occur due to a gathering of like-minded players on a regular basis. Felicity, 76, and Marla, 64, for instance, are on a list for "Thursday Fun Tennis," run by volunteers who book courts, survey availability, and pair contestants.

Sometimes, drop-in play is organized by a facility. This

often happens with pickleball, when a club tries to boost participation by encouraging people to "just show up".

As with golf, these racquet games also support extensive league infrastructure, with national and local organizations that manage competitions.

For tennis, the United States Tennis Association (USTA) works with grassroots entities to create a national ladder of tournaments which moves from city events to sectionals (regional tournaments) to national competition. Several athletes profiled in this book made it to nationals over the years.

Softball is, of course, a team sport played recreationally and in leagues.

Games within games

Those creative ADAPers! A couple of them have jiggled the group format to create games within games. In these, players essentially create new rules for their undertakings.

Doris & Tyrel

On a modest scale, Doris and Tyrel have done this. Theirs is a lively family of sons and grandkids. All revel in games and have made a family tennis tournament a game within a game tradition.

"In the past, we have hosted family tournaments at Thanksgiving," Doris explains. "My youngest is now 6'8" and attended college on a tennis scholarship. But at the family tournament, the older ones will try and get into his head – and they do! Reminds me how mental this game is."

Greta & Charles

For a more extensive example of games within games, consider what Greta, 61, and Charles, 63, have done with golf.

The couple are retired executives who now live in an active golf community just outside Knoxville.

Charles explains, "Greta and I moved here to establish friendships. We went to a yoga class and met a guy who was looking for subs for his couples' group."

Building on this existing arrangement, Greta describes what happened next: "We started 'Kinkaid games', in which each couple hosts the field once a year with a theme [e.g., a current movie, Scottish]. After playing, all participants retire to the hostess' home for a potluck dinner."

They rotate monthly around several courses in the community.

"These are good golfers in Knoxville who want to golf with us. We have 15 couples and eight couple alternates. We had met at our Club, during Friday night mixers and Seinfeld tournaments."

Kinkaid is practical, as well as fun. Comments Charles: "There's almost no on-ramp for non-golfer spouses [who are typically the wives]."

Because the host couple chooses the round format – usually something with a twist - this reduces pressure on the non-player.

For example, the round format could be a scramble with additional rules such as "ladies hit from 100 yards out on numbers 1 and 9" and "pick up from bunker on even numbered holes" and "maximum two putts counted on holes five and 13" and other guidelines designed to reduce pressure.

How format influences satisfaction

Solo athletes may find much satisfaction in the focus they can apply to their undertakings. Plus, they avoid much of the drama and infrastructure demands of team sports.

Team athletes, alternatively, enjoy greater social interactions both inside and outside athletics – this in itself is a major ADAP community satisfier.

The Gamers within Games seek another dimension in their sports. Doris and Tyrel are among the most positive players, so their Thanksgiving "tournament" adds to their pleasure by unfolding the family benefit.

Charles and Greta, on the other hand, have experienced a few more bumps from golf, so their Kinkaid games grew from a desire to compensate for those.

Most ADAPers remain solo or in groups sports, probably more a reflection of how introverted or extroverted they are. If the inward/outward balance is there, the sportsperson is probably positive or somewhat so.

Dimitri

But others, like Dimitri, 62, have shifted.

"Golf is no longer my top priority. I achieve more in endurance sports such as running, swimming. The more I run, the better my time. But practicing more in golf doesn't necessarily lead to dependable improvement.

"Golf is more a believe sport than any other. You have to fall in love with it, but I don't want to be too emotionally wound up by it."

Skill

Not surprisingly, perception of one's skill heavily weights how much an Athlete loves a game (to paraphrase Dimitri).

Belief in one's skill – or lack thereof – is primarily internal. There may be third party opinions, but it's the Athlete's own summing up that matters.

One aspect of this internal skill awareness is *non-comparative*. For example, does the pickleball enthusiast believe he or she has the requisite skill to regularly hit dink shots?

Another aspect of this is *comparative*. Continuing the above example, does the pickleballer have ability to regularly hit dink shots as good as – or better than - all the others with whom she plays?

In a competitive setting, what's the player's assessment of how the relative skills of self and opponent shape the game's outcome?

Finally, does the player believe he or she is moving in the desired skill direction?

How skill influences satisfaction

All these skill aspects and dynamics swirl around in a revolving door inside the ADAPer head. Depending on what exits the door at a given moment, the Athlete will have a good day or a bad day, a love affair or a heartbreak, a confidence boost or a bout of fatalism.

In general, those players whose revolving brain doors allow confidence and optimism to emerge more often than not will be more positive about their playing. They could be at any stage of skill – from beginner to expert – but, in general, the more skilled Age-defying Athletes are *in their own minds*, the more confident they feel, and the more confident they feel, the more positive they describe their game experience.

Skill acquisition *direction* also emerges from the brain's revolving door and influences the player. If a sportsperson believes his or her current skill state is headed for improvement, that person will be less stymied by being at the bottom of the competence ladder, and will be more likely to think positively about the sport.

For another perspective on direction of expertise acquisition, Ivi Kerrigan, Head Tennis Professional at the Hills Country Club in Austin, Texas, advises "...as long as your game is like the stock market, you're doing fine. That is, over time, you will have some ups and downs – winners and losers – but if your playing trend line continues upward, that's quite an achievement."

Noelani

Noelani, a 56-year-old woman who has played pickleball for more than two years, has discovered, "That I pick up things quickly and then I level off. Trying to find ways to move up from this plateau."

Despite this perception of skill acquisition slow-down, she proclaims the game is "a blast. My husband and I feel like kids again. It's not as serious as playing tennis, people don't take it as seriously."

Consistency

Ralph Waldo Emerson once pontificated that

"A foolish consistency
is the hobgoblin of little minds,
adored by little statesmen,
and philosophers and divines."

Most assuredly, Ralph never pitched a curve ball or performed a kick turn.

Otherwise, he would not dismiss consistency as foolish or frightening.

Age-Defying Athletes – irrespective of sport - strive for

consistency. No, not just "strive". They live for it. Dream of it. Cherish it. (And have been known to check the bottom of their elixir tankards for more consistency drops...)

When asked what their late life athletic experience is like, many interviewees in this research initiative express joy, happiness, and pleasure. However, this was frequently tinged with a "But..." that inevitably led to the issue of consistency. As in "But I wish I were more consistent."

Golfers feel more pain about inconsistency than any of the other sportspeople.

Joyce

For example, Joyce, 66, a golfer, addresses the challenge of playing inconsistently with a group of more skilled players.

"I'd like to get to the point to play with LGA [Ladies Golf Association] on a consistent basis ... and understand that it's OK to play at my level and that the ladies don't care how I play," she claims.

"I just don't want to be the worst person," states Joyce. "I want to be good enough not to feel bad that others have to play with me."

Continuing in a philosophical vein, Joyce adds, "It's like a lot of existential goals – shining but moving further away the closer one approaches it... I'm not confident enough for LGA consistently. I really like to play with people who say, 'Just do it again' and then 'See, you can do it!'"

THE ELIXIR OF SPORT

Claude

Claude, 62, notes that a challenge with golf is "How difficult it is to be consistent. The reality of thinking I will hit a wonderful shot now standing over the ball, but then not hitting a wonderful shot. That disconnect doesn't exist in other sports."

Numerous golfers equate consistency with a score.

Shirley

For her golf game, Shirley, a 59-year-old golfer would like "to achieve a low 20 handicap and be able to consistently break 100."

Cormac

Cormac, 62, also has a score consistency goal: "I want to be a bogey golfer, consistently shooting under 90 and at some point, shoot my age…Fewer blow-up holes."

Margot

Even though golfers are those who bemoan inconsistency most often, they don't have an exclusive on it. Margot, a 60-year-old tennis player, for instance, remarks, "I need to improve even more. Need more consistency."

Not surprisingly, inconsistency bedevils those at the Ambivalent end of the spectrum more than either of the other two categories. But it casts a pall for Energized and Muted players, too. And inconsistency is especially galling for any athlete who puts in practice time yet remains, seemingly, at some lousy plateau.

If consistency is so important, why is it so daunting?

The Stages of Learning model offers a clue:

Being inconsistent is part of the learning process. As people progress through the Stages, they overcome rudimentary inconsistencies (e.g., beginner whiffs at a golf ball) and "embrace" higher order ones (e.g., expert who has played the course hundreds of times erroneously reads the back slope of the green for a pitch shot). The inconsistencies are still there, they just become more sophisticated over the years.

Samantha, *The Elixir of Sport* house golf instructor, offers this advice about replacing junior varsity inconsistencies with world-class ones – which is another way of saying that the player is learning:

"Among beginners' most common hitting mistakes are topping the ball, chunking the ball (hitting behind it), and whiffing (swinging without contact).

"Learn to eliminate these and a duffer is on the way up the 'four results buckets':

- Great shots bucket – rare, especially at first
- Good shots bucket – moving toward my goal
- So-so shots bucket – not great or even good, but I can live with it

- Crappy shots (technical term) bucket – topping, chunking, whiffing

"Start by banishing crappy shots and move up to so-so shots. Then reduce or eliminate these so you have mostly good shots. And, finally, wave goodbye to good shots and enter the realm of greatness!"

How consistency influences satisfaction

In general, the more consistent the play, the more satisfied the player. Wishing to improve or "move up" in the game, of course, could balloon inconsistency and transform an Energized ADAPer into a more Muted one. Alternatively, ambition to excel can overcome the downer of inconsistency, plopping the athlete into the Energized zone.

Overall, however, consistency means control, achievement and, not surprisingly, contributes to greater satisfaction.

Competition

For Age-defying Athletes, competition is the 800-pound gorilla in the happy room of playing games.

ADAPers want to play. ADAPers want to win. But back in that corner of that happy room, having a beer and smirking, is Mr. Gorilla. His job is to keep contestants from winning.

Fortunately, that's only half of his job. The other half is

to motivate people to be so good that he cannot possibly perform his task.

Motivation – humiliation. That's the primate's job description. It's demanding for him, but it's profoundly stressful for many players.

Primate management, as many have learned in lengthy non-sport careers, modulates, twists, and turns, as individuals learn more, discard the irrelevant, and embrace the productive.

Over time, ADAP athletes have evolved their relationships with competition, too.

If they regard themselves as competitively successful, they bound toward the Energized end of the satisfaction spectrum. When they run into trouble, they become Muted or Ambivalent. (And timing is everything, as ADAPers can trundle back and forth due to competitive outcomes.)

Competition and gender

Perhaps the most fascinating result of trying to manage the Big Competition Primate is how Age-defying Athlete attitudes toward him tend to coalesce along gender lines.

When ADAP interviewees were asked what they had discovered about themselves by playing a sport, about a dozen of them answered – unprompted – in terms of competition.

Overall, the women seem to have discovered an "I'm here and we're going to deal with this" philosophy for handling the 800-pounder. What's more, for many of them, competition and competition management is a relatively new phenomenon.

The ladies

Clarice

"I know that I am competitive," admits Clarice, an 89-year-old tennis player. "I always knew that I was [competitive] about horses, the piano. I was born that way. I think that's an advantage, because it makes you want to improve... It helps you learn about people. I'm competitive and I try to figure out how to beat my opponents. In life, it's important to develop and use strategy."

Unlike Clarice, however, many ADAP women found vying to be a revelation.

Estrella

Estrella, who is 59 and golfs, describes her competitive awakening. "I'm more competitive than I realized. First year [of playing], I didn't care about winning, and another player told me I needed to complete the scorecard. Now, I'm in it to win it."

Mildred

"I didn't realize I had a competitive streak," notes 73-year-old tennis player, Mildred, "because I had had no prior competitive experience."

Astrid

Competition isn't just about pummeling Mr. Gorilla. Competitive people want affiliation, too, as 88-year-old tennis player Astrid proposes: "I'm competitive and want to be accepted. I like being part of a group, whether I win or not. Having rank is less important than being part of a group at similar level. At the Houston Racquet Club, one would never invite a more highly ranked player to play. There were taboos about skill levels and one did not 'play up'."

Luellen

Some ADAP athletes realize that they are primarily competing with themselves. This is the case for 55-year-old Luellen, a golfer. "I am not as patient as I thought! I am hard on myself. I wasn't competitive with other people, but competitive with myself."

These women appear to be on a relatively even keel with competition.

Other ladies prefer not to punch Mr. Gorilla in the nose,

but, rather, to avoid his corner as much as possible. They compete better when the stakes aren't as high.

Anita

For example, Anita, 78, an avid tennis player states that she is "...nervous in competition, but that's who I am. I don't necessarily play as well in competition as in fun tennis."

The gentlemen

On the Y-chromosome side, it's tempting to conclude that men spent a lot of their early years squaring off with Mr. Gorilla. Today, having little to prove in that battle, they have opted for a hands-off approach.

Female athletes are growing comfortable with their competitive selves. ADAP male athletes are becoming comfortable, too, but with the opposite: with not having to compete as fiercely as they might have in the past. Perhaps their youthful "blood sport" approach to everything from hockey to baseball to football and more has flared out, and now they see other benefits to playing games in later life.

Charles

This attitude is pretty well summed up by linksman Charles: "It's not always about winning. [In contrast] as a youngster, it was always about winning. Golf means support, friends, getting outside, being a little athletic."

Ignaz

The men even go so far as to tolerate not winning. Ignaz, 80, describes his attitude to his tennis game today: "I'm not competitive. I enjoy tennis, but if I lose, that's not a problem. There's a tolerance there…"

Norbert

"I realized I was not as competitive as a lot of guys with whom I play," admits Norbert, another court frequenter. "Sure, I play to win, but losing is not a big deal."

Hudson

Of course, some men wish the Gorilla would leave the room entirely. Hudson, 59, contends "…that I don't like being competitive because it's stressful. Played in a couple of [men's golf league] events. Participants took them very seriously. I want to chill out."

But what about losing?

That's the stressful part of competition, of course. Players have only a limited amount of control over the outcome of a game. And sometimes they lose.

Are renewed selves diminished when players lose? Absolutely not. Renewal doesn't depend on a score. Rather, it's all about being a different person – newer, "younger," more alive - than you were at the start of the game.

The Japanese have a term for this: *ichigo ichie.* Roughly translated as ..."each moment is unique." No moment is shackled to the one preceding it...each is an opportunity to conjure up something beautiful, daring, novel, distinctive, self affirming, bewitching...or to default to same old same old.

Those unique moments are the moments when the potion works its magic. Win or lose, you depart the competition changed from what you were at the start.

Why? Because the very fact that you came out into the light of day to pit yourself against someone who is likely bigger, better, stronger, faster, more skilled, and sneakier (ha!) than you is all that matters.

It's about courage, resilience, commitment – and there you are, an improved version of yourself.

How competition influences satisfaction

Competition is complicated, and in many respects, it's the essence of sport itself.

Certainly, those who win more than they lose will probably inhabit the positive right end of the satisfaction spectrum.

But competition can be neutralized if a player believes he or she is performing well – despite the score.

Competition's influence on satisfaction also can vary

from event to event. For example, if a rower succeeds in a series of events one weekend, that person will likely be more positive about the sport than if she just had just come off a string of defeats.

Regarding competition and gender, it's not that the Energized category is entirely populated by women. But it may well be that more of them popped over there due to a newfound capacity to handle competition.

In similar fashion, the men have morphed into newer, calmer players who greet competition philosophically, and this, in turn, ups satisfaction.

Short-term factors

While frequency, format, skill, consistency and competition are sustained influences in how an ADAP interviewee describes the playing experience, short-term factors also exist. These factors may swing the athlete's sense about a game from positive to negative and back – in the very same day!

Short-term factors include non-personal elements such as playing facilities, commuting distance, availability of playing partners, weather, as well as personal, individual elements like equipment, health, mood (e.g., A soccer player who argued with her husband the night before a match normally would be energized about the game but is distinctly muted about it today.), and more.

Putting it all together, how has the playing elixir effected Age-defying Athletes?

92 ADAP respondents = 92 different perspectives on the sports they play.

But they can be clustered into the three satisfaction categories:

Energized - Most participants were positively charged by their athletic experiences – detailing one or more benefits.

Muted - Interviewees had positive perspectives, but were more subdued about their game playing.

Ambivalent – Some project participants exhibited more "glass half empty" assessments of the experience.

It is important to note, however, that wherever on the spectrum from Energized to Ambivalent an Age-defying Athlete landed, that individual continued playing. Which may suggest that renewal was working its magic even on the more disgruntled Ambivalents?!

Energized

Tyrel

"My tennis life is gratifying," he explains. "It's a huge social thing. We enjoy *apres* tennis as much as tennis. My men's group breaks open a bottle of scotch after our Wednesday evening play [the experience is called Doubles' Doubles].

"I don't need a bigger house. We travel a lot because being a consultant enables working from anywhere on earth. And we play a lot of tennis."

Tyrel, 76, describes a key benefit of the game: "Socialization, talking, being part of a group. Socialization is the #1 thing for longevity, and tennis provides that."

He continues that "Tennis is a pathway to longevity. Doris' [my wife's] Mom played until she was 87, and her stepfather, until he was 92. They were an inspiration.

"I look back at my parents. My Dad died at age 60, and my Mom, at age 75. My father was fit, but he smoked, worked, and bowled. Great sailor and water sports guy. Mom was not particularly healthy last 15 years of her life."

In contrast, Tyrel says, "I feel great."

Perhaps due to the social and physical benefits, he and his tennis buddies do all they can to continue to play. "With our group of men [aged 65 to 83], people get injured – but they always find a way back. They don't want to stop."

Tyrel wrenched a knee snow skiing and was out for three months. He's also had "three heart ablations but those are very temporary."

He is philosophical and notes, "I know I have limitations and we enjoy life."

Vivienne

"Pickleball is the most fun sport I've ever played," declares Vivienne, a petite 70-year-old blonde. "Water skiing is still my favorite, but I cannot ski anymore and we sold our boat. Water skiing is very satisfying when done well. Pickleball is just fun."

She hits the courts three or four times a week. "It's good exercise. Easier on the body than tennis. I've met a lot of new people."

A committed and advanced tennis player, Vivienne got interested in pickleball after her club hosted a pro tournament a couple of years ago. "I attended and it looked like so much fun. Everyone seemed to be enjoying themselves. So I thought 'I should try it.'"

And she wasn't even in the market for a tennis alternative. "I wasn't looking for another sport because I was happy playing tennis."

Nonetheless, she hadn't competed in league tennis for several years, "so I was out of touch except with a small group of [tennis-playing] women."

One surprising aspect of pickleball is that "Men and women play together. Everybody shows up for Friday open play, we mix up and play, friendly to all and welcoming."

Vivienne has discovered "that it's OK to try new things. Normally, I would stick with my regular activities and not step out of my comfort zone. But I did that with pickleball and it's been great."

Her game goal is to play as long as she can and to progress as far as she can.

Luis

Another ADAP participant who is energized by his sport is Luis, 70.

When he was in high school, Luis won a full college scholarship to play basketball.

"I'd played basketball from grammar school through college. And I expected to grow up and become an athlete because I was a lot better than most of my competitors."

Life intervened over the decades, as one might expect, and basketball faded.

Several years ago, he happened to catch a *60 Minutes* program on older softball players competing on teams in Florida. "I said I would do that when I retired."

In the meantime, he had taken up golf. But even though he would hit the links, he hadn't participated in any team sports for decades.

That changed eight years ago, when Luis retired at age 62. Inspired by that *60 Minutes* program, he had been thinking about playing softball for maybe a year, and finally decided to push ahead.

"The difficulty was getting my legs used to running. I wanted to avoid injury. Softball is more sprint like, uses fast twitch muscles."

A self-driving guy, Luis describes how he prepared: "I just went out and started playing. Playing softball is like getting back on a bicycle. Takes time for timing, however."

Expanding about the game, Luis says, "It's Little League for adults who have a lot of fun. [I play on a] formal league in Sarasota, primarily men, about 180 players. Play south

Sota fields from early March until after Thanksgiving, with layover January-February. Everyone plays all season long, no ladder. Games usually in the morning, and some guys drink beer after.

"The camaraderie is surprising. [The league is] competitive, but not too competitive. Surprised by some of the players – one is 78 years old and still runs in Senior Olympics. He's faster than I was in college."

Luis notes the game has benefitted him because "I have a hard time sitting still. Softball keeps me active, outside."

And it's made him realize that he is still very competitive.

He is motivated to improve, and practices a lot. "I hit balls in the batting tee, watch videos. On non-game days, I walk eight to ten miles a day. On game days, probably half that."

But mostly, his goal is "Not to get hurt so I don't have to miss games."

Muted

Vivienne, Tyrel, and Luis are a good representation of the "Energized" athletes in ADAP. They describe their experiences with gusto, enumerating the advantages bestowed on them by their sports.

In contrast, some ADAPers are more subdued and pragmatic about their athletic pursuits. As with the Energized segment, this Muted group includes men and women involved in all sports.

Jacinta

Jacinta, 75, explains that she began playing golf about five years ago, when she and her husband bought a house in a golf community.

"When we committed to buying this house in 2019, I committed to golf."

She says that there was nothing particularly difficult about golf. "But I thought that having to remember 52 things – about my arms and legs and swing and follow through and more – excessive. In swimming, you just get in the water and move your arms and legs. Golf is tricky."

Jacinta plays about three times a week and is philosophical about the game: "At this stage of my life, I am focused on staying outside, being active, enjoying friends, being together with husband, and golf does this."

She notes that she "...cannot be serious at this stage of life...[I] take things with a grain of salt. Frustration cannot keep you from being outside and being active."

Since her husband is a retired service member, "We can play great courses accessible for military. Enables us to enjoy weather elsewhere."

Jacinta adds, "I am not competitive, but there are times when I am – like when I can hit the ball as far as [my husband] can! It's enjoyable and fun to do well. People who are better than I [am] are not going to kill me.

"Our kids are impressed."

She may be muted, but she is also ambitious. Jacinta still wants to improve. "I want to hit straighter and longer.

Continue to build upper body strength. As an older adult, [I know that] walking and upper body strength [are] vital."

Gail

Gail, 63, did not have an extensive sports background growing up. "I only played neighborhood sports...took gym class. I wasn't permitted to play [after school] sports because I had to be home in time for dinner."

Not only was her game-playing childhood rather sparse, but three or four decades had passed – Gail got married, she had sons - with no participation in any sport.

Her husband came from a tennis family, however, and he had played recreationally when growing up. He encouraged her over the years, and, finally, the moment seemed right.

"My husband is preparing to retire, and we are empty nesters," reports Gail. "We needed to do something. I love group activity, and the exercise. Great to do [tennis] as a couple and with other people."

Several years ago, the family moved to New Mexico. They had a lot going on during that first year in the new house. "...it was emotionally challenging. I was ill then, but still kept going to [the club's tennis] Rookie League. I never stopped. It kept my mind off the other things that were bothering me. Once all that stabilized, and my health was good, things were better."

She describes the experience of tennis as "Good...but it has its ups and downs. There's a lot involved. It's a social event. Tennis plays on your psyche, almost as if I'm back in high school dealing with mean girls. I am not attempting to be a pro, just want to play with others who have good habits, and just want to have fun."

Gail has been surprised to encounter player clans. "There are a lot of cliques, but I need to step back. Some of the most cliquish players are very nice women. We all have different goals."

To her, the most difficult aspect of tennis "was having the confidence to hit the ball."

She expands on this idea: "I lack confidence. I try to calm my mind. But when I play others who are better than me, I worry that they will not want to play with me anymore. So I talk to myself and tell myself that I can do it. Try to relax.

"Not performing or losing are always low points for me," Gail states, "but they're never serious enough to make me quit. I just determine that I need to take a lesson to improve something."

After Rookie League, she joined her initial league team. "It was my first time on any organized team, so some challenges, and after the season, we separated."

However, she goes on, "I recently returned to team tennis, and it's been all good, with personalities clicking. I feel that they know where I am at."

All in all, Gail finds several benefits in playing tennis. "It calms the mind, good therapy. Good exercise. Makes you get out there. For newcomers to an area, it's a good bridge."

Her goals are to play more and to have fun. "I want to improve, but not looking to be a [top] team player. Just have fun with the girls, really social.

"I just get up and go. I'm happy to be doing it."

Ambivalent

Players in the Muted satisfaction category note both positive and negative aspects of their games. For those who dwell in the Ambivalent sector, the emphasis tends toward the negative. Not entirely negative, but more shaded than the Muted crowd, and definitely more shaded than those Energized ones.

Luke

Luke's suppressed reaction to tennis these days reflects a sense of resignation. "I quit trying to improve [my tennis game] years ago," reports the 85-year-old.

Nonetheless, he was a tennis pioneer as a kid:

"I grew up in a small town, and boys had to play everything because there weren't a lot of us in high school: football, basketball, baseball, track, tennis," he proclaims. "It was study hall or sports, and I picked sports."

Luke talks tennis: "I didn't know anything about tennis until I was a high school freshman. After our basketball workout one day, our coach directed me and another player outside to our two new tennis courts – both of which had no space along the sides or the back. They ended in gravel. And there were no fences around them either, so we had to chase balls a long way."

"Anyway," Luke continues, "he opened the trunk of his car and pulled out two wooden racquets and announced 'You are our tennis team'. Eventually, there were three of us, but one guy didn't stick with it. We played in an interscholastic league. We were allowed only one can of balls per season."

From that start, Luke continued to make do: "I was self-taught, no lessons or clinics. .... Invented serve which also was invented by someone else and called the American Twist."

He describes the game as an "Important part of my life and I've had good friends and good times. Socially great."

Luke says, "You can play competitively in a match and then stop at the hotel bar for a drink later. Total break and distraction from work."

Some of Luke's muted attitude about tennis may be due to his perception of his physical condition. The low points of the game, he declares, "... were my rotator cuff injuries. Both rotator cuffs injured and required surgery. Right one more serious and I was out for six months. Just took time to heal."

"I'm deteriorating," he concludes, "no longer as athletic as I used to be, but I didn't expect anything different. Just trying to hang on."

Charles and Greta

Charles and Greta value their Kinkaid couples group because both had false starts identifying golf buddies when they moved to the Knoxville area.

Charles recounts: "My first experience was as the 'new person' with a set group [of men] that had played together for years. But they were too focused on the rules. My ball landed next to a tree and there was no way I could hit it without wrapping my club around the tree, so when I moved it, they gave me a hard time."

"Learning the rules and responding to 'advice' are part of the game" he admits, "but I eventually ended up playing with a group of individuals much better than I who give me advice that is tremendously helpful."

Greta relates a similar tale.

"I played a tournament in a member-guest [format]. My partner and I won," states Greta. "I invited her to play at our home course [in another event] and we didn't play well, another nasty experience. The bitch official claimed I had shot a nine on one hole because I whiffed the ball, but it was really an eight."

On another occasion, Greta recalls, "[Charles and I] participated in a tournament and we came in last, horrible experience. The wife of our opponents was not very nice. I moved my ball from behind a tree and she said 'Don't do that.'"

Once they returned to the clubhouse, Greta and Charles learned to their chagrin that the offending couple had placed third.

Ashi

Ashi, 77, started playing tennis in her 30s and now plays once or twice weekly.

It began when Ignaz, her husband, "started playing mixed doubles with a work colleague – a good player. However, Marcia [Ignaz' female colleague] had just married Ricky who didn't play."

Ashi proceeds with the story: "Ricky and I would try to hit the ball over the net on the court adjacent to where our spouses were playing. That's when I started thinking that I liked this. We had fun and I decided to start playing."

Eventually, Ashi and Ignaz joined a tennis club.

Once there, "I was recruited to a USTA team. I told our captain 'I'll do the best I can'. I began doing drills and those were very helpful. Not competitive, just doing the best we could. Our pro was super patient, and I wanted to do a good job for her."

On the team, Ashi says she was blessed with exceptionally fine partners. "We actually went to Sectionals and National."

Despite this achievement, ambivalence always clouded her picture.

She recalls, "I am not competitive, and even though we had that [National] achievement, I always felt that I was the weakest player on the team, and that this was holding us back."

"Additionally," Ashi continues, "my teammates were very competitive and really wanted to win, so I became uncomfortable. At one point, I lost my temper with a dear friend and teammate. So, I knew it was time to retire. This was a very painful decision. It was surely the low point in tennis for me."

Regarding goals for tennis, Ashi continues her ambivalent theme.

"Yes and no on having goals. I want to continue to play with people I like. Also want to continue to learn new things that make me better. Hope no injuries or illnesses keep me from playing. Tennis people have been a real support to me."

Anita

Anita, 78, is a couple-times-a-week tennis player, vying primarily in doubles, with the occasional singles match. She likes the game, but has had a couple of unpleasant surprises.

When she and her husband lived overseas, she reports, "I played singles fun tennis. On this occasion, a woman whom I considered my friend was very cold to me and I felt terrible. Then I realized she was more competitive than I and our friendship changed and that surprised me."

A team experience was similarly an unexpectedly unpleasant one. Anita describes what happened: "Our USTA team out west was cut-throat and [the captain] put me up against our opponents' #1 player, so [our] best player could win, even though I was thrown to the wolves. I was definitely not as serious as others."

Sipping the elixir...

Age-defying Athletes quaff the sports elixir and experience varying levels of satisfaction. Athletes can bounce around the levels over time, but, in general, they tend to hover in the Energized, Muted, or Ambivalent category.

Irrespective of where they land on the satisfaction spectrum, these ADAP interviewees return again and again to play. It's almost as if they become existentially dehydrated and need the nectar of their games.

Each moment is unique, according to the Japanese expression *ichigo ichie*. And every moment when playing – whether the game be sort of OK, mostly positive, or very positive – is a moment these men and women can become new, young, and fresh versions of themselves.

Chapter 6
Benefits of Playing

"The play's the thing..."
—William Shakespeare, Hamlet, *Act 2, Scene 2*

Why do kids like to play?

Partly because they can run around and jump and swing at things and laugh.

Play is their chance to experiment with a new move or game or team or catcher's mitt or swim fins.

Kids like playing because games free them from their quotidien existence and the worries that prey on their minds – school, parents, clothes, personalities, and the eternal question of "Who am I?".

Mostly, they play because they want to have fun.

The elixir of sport is concentrated "kid-ness" (without the bad parts of childhood such as zits, self-consciousness, and Sister Palimpsest).

Playing, play, and play

Besides the use of "play" with respect to games, the word has two other connotations that are relevant here.

There's "play" as in a theatrical production. In a play, people take on novel roles, shedding their day-to-day existence to try on new personas. Actors transform themselves physically, mentally, psychologically, and culturally into new entities. In this way, they liberate their former selves and become new.

Another useful meaning of "play" is the phrase "play on words". In a play on words, a second meaning of a word or phrase brings about a new insight about something. It, too, elevates meaning above the ho-hum.

Like the elixir, and in all these three meanings, "play" is transformational. That's the overall idea.

Peel down a level, however, and it becomes apparent that the benefits of play are the engine that drives the transformation.

Why do adults like to play?

Pretty much for the same benefits kids love: the joy of movement (irrespective of how awkwardly they sashay around), the opportunity to experiment with a new role (athletic, not old), the novelty that comes with sports (win or lose), the feeling of freedom from care (if only for the duration of the game), and being with their friends.

In other words, men and women don new personas as do

actors, and play on their identities (instead of playing on words). In these transformations, they become renewed, reinvigorated, revitalized by sports.

As mentioned in earlier chapters, research with Masters Athletes conducted by Dionigi et al. in the early 21st century found similar results for the effect playing had on elites competing in Masters Games.

The researchers found that many Masters athletes reported that competing in the Games kept them "young". They competed against younger players in many instances. Masters' participation was physically, mentally, and socially important.[26]

Grown-ups emerge renewed by play – even if they have been humiliated and infuriated and drained by it. They are stronger for having participated in a game, and, they are more resilient for returning again and again.

Returning again and again echoes another theme from the Masters Athletes research: players need to hang on because they don't want to lose it.

The studies by Dionigi and other researchers indicated the importance of "not losing it" experienced by these older jocks. "Not losing it" carried a philosophical punch: athletes can still compete in Masters Games, and, by extension, can still compete in life.[27]

Age-defying Athletes circle to their games because of the benefits - friendship, fun, fitness, family connections, fresh air – even winning bets – sure.

But they stick with play because they, too, don't want to "lose it" – however they interpret "it". With "it," they can still compete in life.

ADAPers are hooked on "being out there". Many interviewees describe this benefit along the lines of "It gets me out there." "Out there" could be out of the house, but it could also mean out of a rut, out of what they were yesterday, out to where life happens.

Note that all the benefits arrive irrespective of how well a sport is played. Camaraderie, for instance, develops based on the bond of simply showing up and participating with a group of like-minded individuals. Friendships don't "improve" as one's backhand "improves," in other words. (This doesn't apply to cliques – a diametrically different situation.)

Top-line benefits in the words of Age-defying Athletes

"Huge sense of accomplishment, satisfaction of learning little things, like the transition from one sport to another." – Ling, 56

"I think I let things go a little more [now]. Don't have to win. Happy where I am as I get older. It's OK to lose. Always had to win when younger." – Crawford, 66

"Enjoyment in being outdoors and improving at something difficult. Camaraderie." – Francisco, 79

Achievement, enjoyment, learning, fitness, relaxation, self-acceptance, camaraderie, conquering a challenge, fresh air.

These benefits and more build and reinforce personal rejuvenation. Through playing games, ADAP participants continue to grow and develop as human beings. Some may be developing more in the physical realm, some in the psychic, some in externalities like friendship.

What's more, personal growth and development lead these respondents to reject aging stereotypes. They continue to attempt things that matter to them, irrespective of how society/well-meaning friends/family members view the wisdom of their actions.

Benefit characteristics

For 92 interviewees, the categories of sport benefits span quite a range, from camaraderie to retirement pursuit to travel rationale to mental sharpness to buying cute golf clothes.

The most-cited benefit is friendship, which also incorporates family relationships (usually between spouses, but sometimes between parent and children).

Keep in mind that, as documented in the "Deciding to go for it" chapter, "friendships" was the most frequently cited inducement for *starting* a sport, too. Many of the other benefits discussed in this chapter echo the reasons games were pursued in the first place.

(It's not often in human endeavors that one actually reaches the target at which one aimed, but in sports, that happens.)

The next benefit most often mentioned is physical fitness, followed by mental health, then fun, fresh air, and "being out there".

It's important to note that members of each satisfaction segment described in the last chapter report benefits – even those whose experiences are Muted or Ambivalent.

Many respondents tick off several advantages of play.

For example, Murten, a 59-year-old golfer lists this bunch: "[More] competitive, improved hand-eye coordination, socialization, enjoying club, time spent with husband ..."

Benefits cut across sports – all the team athletes, for instance, claim socialization and fitness advantages. Solo sport gamesters are more likely to focus on fitness, but even a couple of them admit to camaraderie.

The only benefit category that doesn't cut across sports is fresh air – golfers are most likely to resonate to this. The softball player also cited it as did one tennis player who doesn't like to play indoor matches.

Importantly, for golfers, "fresh air and outdoors" aren't merely advantageous phenomena – they are the very core of the game, because golfers are essentially vying against nature. They have to be intimate with it.

Benefit categories in more detail

Embracing friendship

When do people make friends? For most, that happens during childhood. Schools, clubs, churches, neighborhoods, and similar gathering "vehicles" are the most common crucibles for camaraderie.

Friendship-formation certainly doesn't occur much in later life. In fact, a friendship study[28] found that the average age when people meet their best friend is 21.

Thus, Age-defying Athletes probably have not made any

new friends for at least 30 years. Considering the ebb and flow of comrades due to relocations, life changes, and death, the friendship inventory may be pretty low.

ADAP interviewees recognize this. Hence, the significance of building new and rekindling old friendships via playing games.

Many forms of socialization

One form of friendship benefit is *network expansion*. Georgette notes that she "has more friends than I've ever had."

Isaac describes the T for Tennis network interaction, "Social thing is a big deal in tennis. Tennis a good way to nurture friendships. In T for Tennis, Saturday mornings after play, all of us – sometimes as many as 20 people – would go out for coffee. Non-playing spouses would join us. Players would also host parties for us. Great way to get to know each other."

There are the *gender* forms of socialization. For example, Borden appreciates golfing with his "guy friends".

Similarly, Tim notes, "Most of my male friends are from golf."

And Ignaz says, "It's good exercise. Real draw is the camaraderie. Get together with guys to play on a regular basis, chat, have a beer."

And on the female side, "Met most amazing women (I didn't like women pre-LGA.) They were encouraging, loving, and I have made lots of friends," states Luellen.

Another friendship advantage is that it enables *newcomers* to settle into a new community.

As Marla states about tennis, "When you move to new place, people will ask you to play, and you become part of the community...Camaraderie... figuring out their game. I'm always meeting new people. Learn something new each time I play."

Sam and Miriam

New address orientation support was also a plus for Sam, 75, and Miriam, 65, who moved cross country in 2023. "[Pickleball] provided a nice social entrée when we moved here. Miriam never played team sports and now plays doubles."

Sam continues: "We have met a lot of people from neighboring towns. You come into a new community, and pickleball is a great way to meet others. Fun to play, but not fun to lose!"

"The local Food Bank," he reports, "periodically hosts a social open play night in which participants bring food to share plus food for the Bank. There are lots of good things to eat and people have a good time. There's a wide range of ages. Pickleball is like e-bikes – it lets people continue moving who might otherwise not move."

"As medicine gets better, people live longer and healthier," Miriam chimes in. "It's nice that some sport has come along that keeps them moving and socially interacting. Old people can actually do it. Some players are not terribly mobile looking, but they do well. Couple of players in 80s as well as teenagers."

Another form of camaraderie is *deeper understanding of the friends one already has*.

It's not just about acquiring new "play mates," but also about comprehending them more. Explains Aquamarine, "I have learned a lot about my friends, learning their habits. Golf encompasses a lot."

A tarter take on this idea comes from 70-year-old Wilma, a tennis player: "I love the people, even the nasty ones."

Deathracer friends support each other. San Diego is home to a group of older skateboarders called Deathracer413. Their slogan is "One step ahead, one step from dead".[29]

Not promising grounds for cuddliness, but being part of the Deathracer community has been vital to some.

For example, one boarder who survived stage IV throat cancer referred to the boarders as a "lifesaver".

Another who grew up in not-exactly-the-healthiest-of-environments on Venice Beach in California claims Deathracer supported a lifestyle change for the better.

"And that's kind of the point," explains a Deathracer. "It's a huge draw of skateboarding: the community."

The group skates every Saturday, bonding, sharing stories and challenges.

"Skateboarders are all like family," said one 50-year-old who got back into skateboarding five years ago after recognizing something was missing in this life. "It doesn't matter what color you are, what gender you are, it doesn't matter anything. If you roll on four wheels, you're family."

And, for Age-defying Athletes, it doesn't matter what

age you are either, as friendship *crosses age boundaries*. Female tennis player Gudrun claims, "Keeps me younger to be around younger people. What inspires me is being around younger women."

Soloists enjoy camaraderie, too. "I meet guys and kibbitz in the locker room and that's fun" declares solo swimmer Warren. "...Camaraderie. Importance of fellowship and familiar routine. I'm recognized when I go to the balloon pool, feel like I belong, that I'm part of something. I couldn't continue if I swam in an isolated pool; I enjoy being with people."

Tuning the body

As do friendships, the physical fitness benefit covers a lot of territory: weight loss, flexibility enhancement, sleep improvement, no aches and pains, reduced blood pressure, strong back and joints, and "keeps me young and vivacious".

Fitness in the here and now

The fitness benefits of weight loss, flexibility, etcetera, are achieved by Age-defying Athletes in the present, with the promise of continuing into the future as long as playing recurs.

For example, Daisy and Devon describe numerous physical benefits that can be measured and enjoyed today.

THE ELIXIR OF SPORT

Daisy

A 64-year-old tennis player, Daisy ticks off some of the fitness benefits of the game: "Lower cholesterol and blood pressure. It's the best exercise that ever happened to me... Now that we are club members, I can play tennis and also go to gym, do yoga, Pilates. I still walk."

Something that surprises her is that "I could be a good lady athlete. I wish I had started earlier and grown taller!"

Daisy also relishes the comradeship aspect. "I have made friendships, and can go out with friends, to parties, to socialize."

Tennis is "wonderful," she comments enthusiastically.

"It's been good for my relationship with my husband, because now he and I have shared interests. This has grown as I have improved," she asserts. "When we started, I was so bad that it wasn't much fun for him to play with me. But now we are more equal and can compete with each other."

Devon

Devon, a 74-year-old pickleball player, effervesces about the fitness advantages of his new sport. For one thing, his conditioning has improved. For another: "I have lost weight. My appetite has lessened. My brain doesn't say 'get a bag of chips' as much anymore."

Fitness for the long haul

Longevity is another measure of fitness. Unlike weight loss and blood pressure reduction, longevity can only be measured in the future. But the preponderance of evidence is that (a) the physical benefits of cardiovascular improvement and musculo-skeletal health outlined above will support a long and healthy life, and (b) actual studies have demonstrated the positive impact playing sports can have on longevity.

Copenhagen City Heart Study

As far as (b) is concerned, the Danes have been looking into this topic for more than 25 years. In 2021, the Copenhagen City Heart Study, which followed 8577 people those two-and-a-half decades, reported that tennis, badminton, and soccer were the sports that added the most years to human life span.

Tennis led the trio, serving up almost 10 extra years. Badminton packed on an extra six years, and soccer, almost five.

As reported in *Mayo Clinic Proceedings*, the research zeroed in on racquet sports:

"… racket sports[30] appear to be particularly great at increasing life expectancy, due in part to their social aspect, but also perhaps because they are physically challenging and require balance and mental strategy, along with certain visual and spatial elements…"

"And a study of inactive older adults in rural Utah"[31] the

Proceedings article continued, "found that pickleball improved their vertical jump (a marker of mobility) and cognitive performance, and there was a decrease in self-reported pain. Participants in the study also reported a desire to keep playing pickleball even after the study was over."[32]

The Danish study targeted the improved physical benefits of tennis, badminton, and soccer for longevity enhancement.

But another work on US Olympians emphasized disease reduction as a way to stack on more years.

US Olympians study

Maybe it's not surprising that athletes who ascend to the heights of Mount Olympus (metaphorically speaking) live longer.

In this research, former US athletes in either the summer or winter Games between 1912 and 2012 were studied. The result found that they lived, on average, five years longer than the general US population.[33]

The research reviewed the causes of death. Olympians' longevity was primarily due to lower rates of cardiovascular disease and cancer than experienced by the general population.

Additionally, lower rates of respiratory diseases, accidents, homicides, endocrine and metabolic diseases, and digestive system diseases also contributed to those extra five years.

Interestingly, however, the US Olympians and the general population did not differ on mental illness and nervous system disorders. The human brain is powerful. The Olympians' presumed ability to focus and excel despite having brains that flipped and flopped like the rest of humanity adds extra dimension to their achievements.

The Olympian research appears to confirm compression of morbidity. Compression of morbidity is the concept that an individual lives a more or less consistently healthy life until the very last second, then pops off to that arena in the sky.

As the Olympians research indicates, the physical, psychic, and social benefits of games can greatly promote compression of morbidity.

What about golf?

With these results about racquet sports, soccer, high jumps, sprints, swimming, and all the rest, should golfers toss their clubs into a handy water hazard?

(This is reminiscent of the superb opening scene from *The Philadelphia Story* in which Katherine Hepburn breaks ex-hubby Cary Grant's golf clubs over her leg. Either those hickory shafts were very flimsy back then or her quads were karate calibre!)

Golfers, don't despair: Hang onto those sticks. Another Scandinavian study, this time one from Sweden, found that golfers also enjoyed about five extra years of life.

According to the R&A (Royal & Ancient): "Published in the *Scandinavian Journal of Medicine and Science in Sports*, a landmark study found a 40% reduction in mortality rates among 300,000 members of the Swedish Golf Federation, corresponding to an increase in life expectancy of about five years (this applied for both genders, all ages and all socio-economic groups)."[34]

None of these studies cover the quality of that augmented longevity, but it's probably a solid guess that the longer time is a continuation of the prior healthy years.

Currently, no information is available about the longevity impact for other sports not studied, but, by extrapolation, they will probably come up pretty well.

Doris

Doris, 76, did not participate in many sports when she grew up. "I was kind of a nerd, the oldest of five, and 'the unathletic one'. I was more interested in theatre, debate. In college, I took standard PE classes."

"My mother was an inspiration to me, however," Doris continues. "She played high school tennis, then took it back up later in life and played until she was 86. She was married three times and her third husband played until he was 95. They were very tied into the greater Miami tennis scene.

"My mother would sometimes hit tennis balls in the street with me when I was growing up, and sometimes I would hit balls against a wall, but this was nowhere near 'playing'."

As an adult, Doris "kind of fell into" tennis at age 53. "When my youngest was in the fourth grade, I took him to tennis lessons at our club. There was another mother there doing the same thing. So I thought that rather than sit in our cars awaiting our sons, we might as well try it ourselves."

Given her childhood emphasis on non-athletic pursuits, it's probably not surprising that Doris remarks, "I'm not an exerciser, so [tennis] is my exercise. I'm a social exerciser, so I probably could walk and talk, but I play tennis.

"After tennis, I tell myself, 'Physical activity – check'."

She also reminds herself that "we are not the athletes we thought we were ten or even five years ago."

Ironically, however, Doris has discovered "...that I'm reasonably athletic. One of my sisters has gone back to pickleball, and the other one is a regular walker. But I'm the only one who followed Mom."

The 76-year-old has formulated no particular goals for her game, other than to say, "If it stops being fun, I will quit. Sometimes you play so badly you want to burn your racquet, but you still come back."

She came back following significant physical challenges, too. "Yes, breast cancer with radiation treatment was long ago and I was out for that. I also ran over my leg with my husband's truck and was in a boot for awhile. In both instances, I just came back and started playing again.

"Whenever someone is out, they worry about losing muscle tone and playing ability, but I just got over that."

Anita

Another longevity enthusiast, Anita, declares, "So many ways [have I benefitted from tennis]. To stay fit, have to be serious about activity."

"Years ago," she relates, "I read a *Time* magazine article

that a physically fit person would live independently ten years longer than an unfit one.

"I had no kids of my own," Anita continues, "so I had to be independent. *Younger Next Year*[35] [is a book that promulgates] if you exercise 45 minutes per day [the] body will 'believe' it is being active and healthy and stay active and healthy to support that."

Because of this, Anita says playing sports means "...you get to have fun as well as be active. Social friendship - just to have group of friends. Fun relationships that are meaningful but not necessarily reliant on conversation."

The Masters Athletes research[36] also circled around longevity, primarily due to the emphasis participants placed on youthfulness. For the majority of Masters participants, "the satisfaction of knowing that [they were] not losing it"[37] was extremely important.

In other words, by monitoring their performance in the context of sport, the participants demonstrated that "I can still do it [i.e., compete]! I'm not too old."[38]

Defy age and live longer

ADAP respondents would be impressed by the long life statistics. One of their primary goals with respect to the ticking clock is to "just continue to play as long as I can."

Hazel is 76 and is a polysport, frequently found on both the golf course and the tennis court.

Here's what she says about lifespan and play: "From what I notice, those who play tennis live longer. They move.

Socialization. Thinking is enhanced, have to remember scores. It's camaraderie, exercise, mental."

Then she laughs and adds, "I'm a stupid kid again." Tennis is a "lifetime sport that I never thought I would still be [playing] at age 76."

"I look at [82-year-old] Phyllis, [77-year-old] Ashi, [83-year-old] Mona, and they are an inspiration to me," comments Blair. "Being active is key to aging well."

82-year-old Phyllis herself notes that "I don't want to quit [playing tennis]. I like to play. I like the ladies with whom I play and plan to play until I am 95."

And for a pragmatic opinion about playing tennis in later life, there's Norbert: "At my age, my goal is not to fall down while on the court."

Tuning the brain

Mind improvement from playing games is one of the most surprising findings from the ADAP research.

What?! Old people improving their cognitive function?

That goes against the grain of 3000 years of civilization, in which old people were pudding heads plodding toward their recliners in the stars.

Civilization is wrong on this one, because Geezer brain renewal happens, as the Age-defying Athletes Project proves.

Participants describe the psychic benefits in terms such as "mentally, I'm still young," and "strategy good for brain," and "mind taken off worries," and "sense of purpose," and "focus, live in moment".

THE ELIXIR OF SPORT

Nate

Growing up, Nate, 73, played all sorts of sports: football, baseball, track through high school. He even took tennis lessons in junior high, but didn't keep at it.

What he did continue with was basketball, which he played until he was 45.

Yes, into his mid-40s. While he was still working, Nate even played basketball during lunchtime.

He never expected to be an athlete as an adult, but, unfortunately, he suffered athletic injuries.

"I lost both ankles playing basketball and wish I'd quit earlier and started tennis sooner."

He totaled three ankle replacements, "...and took ten weeks off for each. But I was able to come back surprisingly fast. [Ankle] replacement is simple, so as soon as the replacement was set and calcified, I was back."

Then, new ankles and all, "I was transferred for my job and there was no basketball at lunchtime, which was what I had been used to. But there were industry events around tennis, especially doubles, and there was a lot of camaraderie."

So, that's how Nate began playing tennis.

He is a keen observer. "I can always tell people who played since they were kids. Their strokes are strong and dependable."

For Nate, the prime benefit of playing tennis is that it both calms his mind and keeps it sharp.

The game provides "...mental relaxation. Mentally very relaxing to keep score. I don't care who wins or loses (much!) but the process of keeping score helps me focus on the game. That's why I like competitive sports."

Another cognitive angle is that "As I play better, I have more fun. Then strategy enters the game. The mental part is where I can pick up on weaknesses in my opponents, and then exploit those weaknesses."

His goal is to become more consistent so he can enjoy more of this psychic benefit.

Probably because he thinks deeply about the game, Nate notes, "I am also surprised that more people don't analyze, they just go through the motions. I can tell what their first two shots will be…very predictable."

He is surprised "that more people don't play, given the mental, conditioning, and friendship benefits."

Blair expands on some of Nate's commentary about how sport strengthens players mentally.

This 62-year-old tennis player professes, "I like orderliness, etiquette, clear rules, friendliness, sportsmanship. These are all parts of tennis."

Somewhat piquantly, given her husband's avidity about golf, "I like that you have done something that can be accomplished in two hours vs. more than double that time for 18 holes."

Have fun - again

"Fun" is a funny word. It connotes lightheartedness, but it encompasses the deeper pleasures that make life worth living: joy, delight, merriment, diversion, laughter, even battle of wits ("You're funning me…").

And, of course, kids equate playing with fun.

Can grown-ups really have fun? There are certainly any number of Schools of Thought which propound that fun is impossible for the senior set. So, having fun (and being proud of it) is another way of thumbing the ancient nose at aging stereotypes.

Francisco, 79, sums up the physicality and sociability of fun: "[It's the] sheer joy of smacking a golf ball on the screws on a pretty day with your buddies."

Some Age-defying Athletes are inspired by the fun they see in others. For example, Marla was drawn to tennis because "I just saw a lot of women playing and it looked like fun."

Nowadays, she adds, there is no need for a reason to hit the courts. "I am always motivated. When I see my racquet, I know I will have fun."

Often, fun is a label for a bushel of virtues. "I meet new people...love the social aspect," Leslie, 64, affirms. "It's competitive, but friendly. Pickleball sorts itself out by rotating after each game, so people eventually end up playing at their level. I think it's fun out there. Always playing a game is fun."

A fun sport is also great in comparison to other fitness activities, as Audrey, 62, asserts. "Tennis challenge keeps me coming back. It's cardiovascular fitness. Really been fun, not a grind like riding a spin bike."

Fun is a popular ADAP benefit, but it's also a goal for a number of Age-defying Athletes.

Mildred is a proponent of fun as a goal. This tennis player contends that, "I will continue to play as long as I can and have fun, but I don't expect to become a 4.0 [rated player]."

Lack of fun is also a motivator for some. "I was not getting anywhere [with her golf game] and that wasn't fun," reports Betje.

She changed from a traditional golf instructor to a high tech training facility that enabled her to view her swings. "I am a visual learner," she continued.

Again that kid thing. Betje adds, "I discovered that I was able to get better [after lessons] and that I wished I'd played as a kid."

Freshen in fresh air

Being outdoors, in fresh air, surrounded by nature is an important benefit and motivator – especially for golfers.

McGregor, 86, took up golf because he "Wanted to be in the fresh air, walking."

Natasha, 80, confirms the power of the outdoors in the overall golf experience. "Making friends. Social part I like. Get out, exercise, fresh air, play with [my husband]."

It's also a great motivation for her: "Some days I have to tell myself that we might as well go out and get some fresh air."

Leon, another 80-year-old golfer, ticks off links benefits: "Friends. Fresh air. Pleasant experience. Lovely courses."

However, this one-time expert bowler (think indoors) asserts that those same natural beauties create a complex sport. "Golf is way more difficult than bowling. Lies, heavy grass, reading greens, on and on and on."

Brett votes for the outdoors, as well. Golf's advantages,

he notes, are "Social, great way to meet a lot of different people. Fresh air, physical exercise."

Be "out there"

Being "out there" means not being "in here"...not sequestering at home, not protecting oneself with the tried and true, not hiding within an old self.

Many respondents – both men and women – used the expression to capture different aspects of play. Often, it meant that they were letting go of the need to control. Sometimes "out there" meant exposing oneself as not being particularly athletic. For others, "out there" was simply about having something to do.

Ramona describes the tendency to self-protect with respect to golf. "Most difficult [aspect of golf] was the mental part of putting myself out there and wanting to do well. I took it so seriously. Perfectionist."

Betje interpreted the term slightly differently: "Golf is a good way to meet people, keep in shape. Keeps you 'out there'."

Carmella, a Prodigal, says about tennis that "The most difficult aspect was just playing the first real match, and putting myself out there to meet people."

For all of the Age-defying Athletes, play is not only a physical phenomenon, but it's a reason for getting up in the morning, for paying attention to date and time and people and seasons.

64-year-old Wanda, a golfer, notes that the game is "a

good way to meet people, keep in shape. Keeps you out there - otherwise, I would sit in my sewing room all day long, closed in on myself."

Elixir is concentrated "kid-ness"

For older adults, sports are rejuvenating – they make Geezers young again. Sports reinvigorate friendships, physical health, mental acuity, fun. Games connect athletes with nature and the outdoors. Above all, sports turn players inside out so that newer – if older – versions of them emerge "out there".

There's a certain closure, as well, with these benefits. Most of them were also the reasons that ADAP respondents decided to play sports in the first place, with friendship, fitness, and fun topping the deciding factors list.

Chapter 7
Discoveries & surprises

"The real voyage of discovery consists not in seeking new landscapes, but in having new eyes."
—*Marcel Proust,* La Prisonniere

Discoveries unlock potential

Columbus discovered the western hemisphere and unlocked the potential of that land mass for the rest of the world.

Penicillin was discovered by Alexander Fleming in 1928, thus unleashing the potential of antibiotics that have saved millions of lives in the century since.

While Sir Isaac Newton didn't precisely discover gravity, he developed the laws of universal gravitation and motion, enabling the potential of physics and the inventions and advances it has fostered.

Discoveries also unlock potential in people who play sports in later life. While these may not be as metaphysically stunning as the world-shattering accomplishments of Columbus, Fleming, or Newton, they are equally as powerful for Age-defying Athletes.

What is this potential? It comes from the elixir and is the potential to be new again, revitalized, refreshed – even if only for the morning pickleball match or afternoon spent in the pool.

What "new" looks like will vary with each Age-defying Athlete. Maybe the revitalization is in some physical realm, such as improved coordination. Or perhaps it's more in the relationship realm, with the pleasure of friendships that did not exist six months ago.

Even more amazing, these refreshed and rejuvenated men and women are well past the age when – according to conventional views of aging – they should have expected anything like that to happen.

Add a new dimension to that Geezer brain to solve a strategy problem on the tennis court? Yup.

Recognize that the insight about "my self-confidence has increased" is the first new insight one has had in a decade? You got it.

Renew loyalty and love of important values such as achievement, courage, self-acceptance? Ditto.

All these and more potentials are unlocked by the seemingly simplistic act of moving through space, frequently in opposition to or in coordination with others.

ADAP participant discoveries and surprises

What did Age-defying Athletes discover from playing?

As with all things related to ADAP, many respondents were over-achievers: they discovered several things and had a number of surprises.

Naturally, there were outliers, as a few didn't discover anything about themselves! However, they learned unexpected things about the game, equipment, or other players.

All in all, ADAP responses coalesce around five themes of self-discovery and surprise: achievement, problem solving, transformative emotions, athleticism, and other players and quirks.

Achievement

Irrespective of whether they are Sports Virgins, Prodigals, or Continuers – or Ambivalent, Muted, or Energized - ADAP respondents often cite "achievement" as a discovery or surprise. They have realized that they can play a game, that they can succeed at it, that a part of life previously inaccessible to them is, indeed, at their fingertips.

As might be expected, the keenest sense of accomplishment surprise is reserved for Sports Virgins who are pleasantly shocked by what they can grasp.

Aquamarine

For example, recalling when she began, Aquamarine declares she is surprised "...that I can actually [play golf]! Starting a foreign sport could have been overwhelming. I just practiced and practiced because I wanted to succeed and hold my own. If we succeed and hold our own, we are winners."

Aquamarine took up the game about nine years ago "basically so my husband and I could do something together."

Married to an enthusiastic outdoorsman, she tried hiking at his encouragement. "...but I didn't like it. We did strenuous hikes, for example, in New Zealand, but it wasn't for me."

In the beginning, golf didn't seem to be for her, either. For several years, "...I rode with my husband in a golf cart at the course near our summer home. This helped me get used to the lingo, the different personalities. My husband was my coach for many years."

She reports that "The most difficult [part of starting to golf] was getting over the fear that everybody was watching me and that they were making fun of me. At the driving range, I worried what people were thinking."

Her natural competitiveness, however, helped her overcome her fretting. "I'm a competitive person, so [golf] plays to that."

Aquamarine has met "great people" and ranks these friendships higher than the physical benefits of the game.

In addition to making new friends and deepening her understanding of existing ones, Aquamarine states, "Golf encompasses a lot. I have learned to ask for help, which is not easy. It's good to ask for help."

Her goal is "Keep playing as long as I can. Just want to enjoy the sport and stay healthy. Play through my senior years.

"You don't have to be the best golfer," Aquamarine asserts, "just get out there and play."

Iolana

"Just get out there and play" could also apply to Iolana, a 76-year-old golfer whose own doggedness was a revelation. "That I stuck with it [was a surprise]," she explains.

Perhaps that's not as unexpected as it seems because she also has discovered "That I can surprise myself with my game, and that I am not a very good judge of what I can and cannot do!"

A one-time expert downhill skiier, Iolana is motivated because "I have a good attitude toward it. When I play poorly, I feel like I'm on a bunny slope, and when I play better, I feel that I have graduated to a green slope."

Nonetheless, she is realistic: "I know I will never be good at [golf], but I like the ladies with whom I play, being outside. All about my attitude. And no one is dependent on my performance, a truly individual sport."

Gigi

Gigi's self-discovery was also about doggedness – but in a broader context. "I learned life lessons from playing [tennis]," this long-time racquet player notes. "So many times, I wanted to quit, but it has taught me resilience. Keeps me young in both brain and body."

Remaining mentally sharp is partially due to how she analyzes tennis: "Doubles is like a chess match with pieces constantly moving. If you miss one, your best shot is your next shot."

She is surprised both by how difficult tennis is as well as by her own athletic accomplishment. Gigi has discovered "That I'm quite athletic. Honestly, I am surprised by that."

Meredith

Golf is difficult, and Meredith, 71, had a goal "When I came here, I wanted to prove to myself that I could go out and play without my husband or my [links expert] mother-in-law, with just a group of women. That I could perform club selection, read greens, and the rest. And I have achieved that."

Self-discovery also included a renewed commitment to commitment itself for Meredith: "I learned that I can be more committed to this than to other things in the past. I don't want to let down friends who are expecting you to play, and don't want to let myself down."

However, she clarifies: "I didn't expect it to be that hard.

But once into the tiny aspects of it – like how to line up a putt – it draws you in. It's easier to learn when younger. But I have stuck with it and have improved. Never tried anything as hard as golf."

Problem solving

Mastering "tiny aspects of a sport"...figuring out a "chess match"..."stepping out of my comfort zone" all reflect problem-solving discoveries made by ADAP respondents.

Here's another one: Warren solves a counting problem.

Warren

Anyone who has ever swum laps knows the headache of keeping track of the number of laps completed. Numerous counting devices are available, but none really worked for Warren, a swimmer in his 70s.

"[The pool's] lane lines used to have beads that helped me keep count [of laps] in sets of five. When the pool installed new lane lines, no more beads. So now, I move clothes pins on the pool deck in groups of five. If I still lose track, I tend to round up!"

Turns out initiating swimming solved another problem for Warren.

"I retired in my mid-50s and started to think that I would become a slug if I did nothing," he recalls. "So, I began walking purposefully through about 2007. But I'm not an athlete and my knees started to ache. I knew walking long distance was not in my future."

Warren continues describing how he solved his conundrum: "By this time, I was 65 and wondered what could I do? I was intrigued [by swimming] because our daughters had been competitive swimmers."

Besides his spectator's appreciation of the sport, Warren liked the idea of less and tear on his joints, too.

"Our town has a balloon pool and I wandered over there in 2012 and thought I may swim."

The facility is an enclosed ("balloon") pool that is 25 yards long, with water heated to 82 degrees.

He reports that it was "slow going at first". But after three to four months, he worked up to 18 laps.

Nowadays, "I do 25 yards free style out, grab the wall, breathe, then do back stroke back."

His results have been substantial – and renewing! "I lost a 'sizable' 30 pounds," he reports proudly. "There's a warm glow of completing activity and swimming renewed that. There's a sense of accomplishment."

In so doing, he discovered "First thing, sense that physically good shape, accomplished, not a slug."

Warren swims solo, but describes ample opportunity to interact with others. "I meet guys and kibbitz in the locker room and that's fun. Camaraderie. Importance of fellowship and familiar routine. I'm recognized when I go to the balloon pool, feel like I belong, that I'm part of something. I couldn't continue if I swam in an isolated pool; I enjoy being with people."

Despite all these benefits, he admits, "Swimming is something I do to keep in shape, but I'm not passionate about it. It's sort of a regular task. I'm not excited about the prospect of swimming, but afterwards, I like it."

He has solved this motivational problem by discovering a natatorium dream: "Paired my fantasy about my swimming with the reality. I fantasize about competing, and that makes my laps go faster."

Warren adds, "If I don't swim three times weekly, I am surprised at how quickly I can build back up again. I tell myself 'just do 15 laps,' but then I find it's easy to complete 18."

Marla

A tennis player, Marla shares Gigi's perspective that playing doubles is like solving chess problems.

"I think of tennis as a chess board and for me it is mentally fatiguing. What is my opponent going to do with that shot? Figuring that out."

She does admit, however, that "I think sometimes I'm hard on myself, second guessing."

"Everyone wants to be the best, get an A. When older, able to focus more, but still want that A. Form of competition – competing against self."

Another problem to solve is the tension between the kinship of playing and wanting to best those "kin". Marla says, "I don't want to make someone feel bad with a great shot – but satisfaction of a great shot suffices."

She values camaraderie, but notes that a benefit she enjoys is "figuring out their game."

Although Marla had an exercise background, she hadn't played many sports before taking up tennis at age 51. "Difficulty? I had never done any racquet sport. Never put something in my hand to hit a ball. All of it was challenging."

She reports, however, "Hand-eye coordination improved. I can now lob stuff into the trash!"

For Marla, problem solving discovery plus achievement discovery.

Another surprise was analytical: "When I watch tennis on TV or go to tournaments, the amount of technique involved is amazing. So much technique involved. Never master the sport but learn all the time."

Delphine

Problem-solving requires focus, as tennis-playing Delphine, 71, discovered. "When I focus, I can accomplish things."

She adds that she has to "concentrate a lot for my age. I have to move. Really improved over the years – practice and play. I take a lesson periodically to check that I am still doing things correctly."

Ashi

In similar focus vein, Ashi states about tennis: "I learned that sport is more than doing activity, it's problem solving. You have to pay attention to what's going on."

She describes herself as "not athletic". Nonetheless, she has renewed herself by becoming a player of sport.

Ashi continues: "I discovered that I can learn to do better. Takes a long time to learn enough to support other players."

Transformative emotions

Games generate an ocean of emotion. Kids games, collegiate sports, adult competitions, pro sports: for players, coaches, and spectators, games are roller-coasters of feeling. Good, bad, ugly. Sort of OK, mostly positive, very positive...

This wasn't just discovered, nor is it surprising.

What certainly has surprised Age-defying Athletes is that emotion can also be transformative. They have discovered that emotion causes them to stop and think about what they are feeling and how it impacts their performance and experience.

This has enabled them to discover insights about their own emotions and how to handle them. A renewed person emerges, this time metamorphosized by emotion.

Brett

Brett, who is in his 60s and has played golf on and off for almost half those years, discovered: "I have learned to put bad shots behind me. I have learned that in terms of controlling my emotions, I have to tell myself that [bad shot] doesn't effect me."

When growing up, he participated in numerous sports – little league, competitive snow skiing, competitive water skiing, track, cross country.

Brett played a little recreational golf with his father, but "I always had the attitude that golf was a game I could always master when older, later in life. But now, I regret that I didn't take it up as a kid. Shouldn't have been on the track team, but golf team instead."

Fast-forward from childhood 20 to 30 years, and Brett is too time-pressed by a demanding career and family responsibilities to participate in athletics.

However, by his mid-50s, he finally decided the time was right to get serious about golf.

"The difficulty was ... the embarrassment of a god-awful slice and the dread of playing with good golfers."

Brett is surprised by the game's fickleness. "It's unpredictability...Difficulty of the game. Every day is different."

Perhaps another emotion he has begun to understand is the contrast of golf with past athletic success – as well as the slipperiness of consistency: "There's the technical difficulty of mastering a skill. I picked up skiing right away, but not golf. Difficult to maintain consistency."

Felicity

Unearthing some fact about emotion isn't limited to the negative feelings such as frustration and embarrassment. Another area of emotional discovery is surprise at liking a game.

In her 70s, Felicity has played tennis since she was 40. She is surprised by "...the fact that I do like it so much. I have several sisters, none of whom play tennis. They cannot believe that I play."

More broadly, Felicity is also "...surprised that I like exercise that much. When I was growing up, no one 'exercised'. We did a lot of outside work such as washing windows, gardening, but nothing that would be considered 'physical' today. Nothing to get the heart rate up."

Hae

Another ADAP respondent surprised by her positive feelings toward a new sport is Hae, 72, "I never thought I would like [golf] as much. It's addictive."

This compliment is quite an achievement in itself, because it comes from a woman who was a ranked amateur tennis player in her youth and who spent much of her career in an allied industry.

Hae started golfing in her early 40s and believes that "You can play golf by yourself and learn about yourself. Very individual sport. Nobody cares what you shoot, just keep up."

Nonetheless, she continues, "You find out that you can get upset. Need to be honest about your score. Years ago, [my company] would take a job candidate out to play to see how he or she did on the course."

Glace

"I have discovered how fun [tennis] is," declares Glace, 61. "There's a lot. Constantly learning and so many things."

Her enthusiasm is balanced by another emotion, however. "I get in my head and that's a downer, and then my game falls apart. Doing well, then I make mistake on mistake. My partner is reliant on me and I don't like letting that person down."

She wants to solve her concentration problem: "Unfortunately, I lose focus quickly."

Davis

Another Age-defying Athlete who found emotional satisfaction through a game is Davis, 51.

"I discovered that I can be happy on the course."

He continues, "[There is a] sense of excitement hitting any clubs, swing coming naturally. [My pro] knows how to teach. Surprise of a good swing, I guess."

Athleticism

"...a good swing...excitement hitting any clubs..." ...athleticism writ large.

The ADAP world revolves around sports and physicality, so one may have anticipated that discoveries about athleticism would be fairly consistent across the Athletes.

Not so. Some discovered that they were athletic, others discovered that they weren't!

Murten

For example, Murten, a golfer, reports: "Surprising when I hit it well. More athletic than I thought."

Another surprise she has experienced is that "I enjoy it more than I thought."

"We have lived in a golf community since 2018," Murten continues. "My husband played golf. Kids were grown. I had the time and energy to learn. Good together as we retire."

Murten enjoys the competition and "feels my hand-eye coordination is better."

"I'm improving - 48 [handicap] to 42," she says. "I've learned to appreciate the game, see value in driving range. Enjoyed and got first time competitive."

Golf is "very honest" and a "true testament to improvement."

For these reasons, the game is rewarding. Of course, in line with a recurring ADAP theme, she would liked to improve faster.

Ling

Another surprised athlete, Ling, 56, a marathoner and triathlete, discovered that "I could be more of an athlete than I thought. That I accomplished this surprised me."

Ling elaborates: "My own grit surprised me. I'm like a dog with a bone, and don't give up even if the going gets tough. I am really competitive. Will fight with someone to beat them.

"I was surprised that the more I practiced swimming, the greater became my determination not to be beaten."

At age 33, following the birth of her second child, Ling decided she needed to lose weight.

"I put on my running shoes and started," she reports, because she didn't want to go to the gym.

But a friend told her that weight loss wasn't a good enough goal, and suggested something else, such as distance. "So, I ran a 5K, then an 8K, and worked up to half marathon. Ran with a lot of training groups, then joined [a] school of running...all different levels."

There's a lot about athleticism that Ling has learned from her experience. For one thing, athleticism is not one size fits all. "All shapes and sizes of people compete in marathons and triathlons."

She notes that "I loved marathons for awhile, but got bored and turned to triathlons. Did one and loved it. Proud that I finished above average for my age group. Triathlons take a lot of time and focus, lots of concentration."

Her athletic discoveries drilled down to specific aspects of the sport. "I learned that I liked cycling, the technology, how to be aerodynamic. Better to use low gear and go slowly uphill than trying to stay in high gear. I learned how to take switch backs."

THE ELIXIR OF SPORT

Patrice

By contrast, tennis player Patrice, 53, learned that "I am not as athletic as I thought I was. Tennis tears you down, so you have to be humble. Exciting and frustrating."

She had not participated in team sports growing up and was only motivated to try tennis because her wife "became a maniac about it." Patrice began three years ago.

A surprise for her was "One reason it's a great game is that there are different levels. No matter how bad you are, you can find someone to play with you."

She comments, "Kids soak things up. But really hard to learn as an adult. Body motion predicated for tennis was not natural or instinctive for me. Plus, adults care more about mistakes."

All in all, Patrice says, she doesn't need motivation to play. "But if I never was improving, that would be different. I am noticeably improved vs. six months ago."

Devon

The athletic discovery for Devon, pickleball player in his 70s, was "How poorly my legs were in running."

He says he played basketball and track in school, plus indoor racquet ball post-education out West. "But I needed to bring my legs up to par [for pickleball]. Racquet ball paddle is close to pickleball paddle, so my brain could eventually determine where to hit the ball."

Devon began playing the court game about a year and a

half ago. Why did he choose it? "I wanted a more athletic sport than golf. Always enjoyed racquet sports and football. Hand-eye coordination. I liked pickleball from the get-go."

Another of Devon's interesting discoveries is that "when you play a sport with several others – such as pickleball – you need to act like a nice person. It's motivated me to up my 'sportsmanship-ness'."

Maybe another reason that he sought a links alternative? "Pickleball players have a lot of fun. There will always be a few grumpy guys and gals, but for the most part, people cheer each other on. Not a lot of golf cheerleaders."

Other players, quirks

As Devon's story illustrates, Age-defying Athletes are keenly aware of others –teammates, competitors, instructors, innocent bystanders – and have revelations about them.

They also have identified quirks about the games themselves.

Tim

Tim, 77, has played golf for almost 60 years. His surprise? "At my age, the thing I most enjoy is that I can compete with people who are younger."

He has discovered that he is "...not as good as I used to

be. Handicap is close to where it used to be, but I don't hit as far as in the past."

"Most of my male friends are from golf," Tim opines. "I am now the old guy. Sport is fun."

It may be a fun game, but as with all human interaction, there has been some "indigestion".

Here's what Tim experienced: "I used to play with the MGA [Men's Golf Association], played in every event they had for a decade. I was one of the top five to ten guys for years in that group. But I had to stop playing with them for reasons that will not be detailed."

Aquamarine

Aquamarine made a similar unsettling discovery, also around links play.

"I tried to get on a nine hole team years ago, but one team member was very critical of me, essentially bullying me," she recalls.

"I came home in tears and lost my confidence."

Over time, Aquamarine put this poor sportswomanship behind her. "Eventually, I met a group of ladies and we just played socially – they are young enough to be my children! They urged me to come back to the team, so I took the bull by the horns and did."

Aquamarine adds a note of poetic justice: "The player who bullied me eventually moved on. And the group now is supportive for all – everyone pulling for everyone else."

Bullying, being poor sports, whining, criticizing, misrepresenting plays, cheating, and worse are part and parcel of sports, of course. They are the dark sides of games.

Doris

And while these may be unhappy truths to discover, they add grit to Age-defying Athletes, such as tennis player Doris.

"I'm surprised by people and what they say and do," she asserts. "Some are such poor sports."

Doris describes a recent match when "Our team walked off the court to reset the score when the other team called 'that [ball] was out'. Our team noted that the players should have made the call at the time, not once the game had ended."

The other team wouldn't let go. Doris continues, "Then later in the match, there was another disagreement, and our opponents commented that 'Well, playing by your rules…'"

Dee

Finally, a discovery about a quirk of golf made by Dee, 82, who began her links play about 15 years ago.

She is surprised by "How many golf balls I can find. And how many people specifically hunt for balls when not playing."

"Our house," Dee explains, "is on a hole with a creek, and every couple of days, we see people trying to retrieve balls from it. Two guys spent about 20 minutes just walking along the creek with ball retrievers the other day. A woman came by later, too."

Discoveries and surprises unlock potential - and potential can lead to invention

There is a story that used to make the rounds at GE about the invention of Lexan® in the 1950s. As the myth goes, a GE scientist was leaving for the day and forgot about a clear substance on a lab bench. He left the compound in a beaker with a test tube sticking out and headed home. When he returned to the lab the next morning, he discovered that the substance had hardened almost to the strength of steel, so much that he couldn't remove the test tube. This eventually became the polycarbonate plastic Lexan.

Age-defying Athletes certainly don't need to spend the night in a lab in order to invent unexpected versions of themselves! Rather, they can count on simply being surprised to discover things about their achievements, problem solving ability, transformative emotions, athleticism, and, yes, even about other players and quirks.

Such novel insights flow from the elixir of sport and unlock Athletes' potential to re-invent themselves.

Chapter 8

Injuries

When the sport beverage is more white lightning than magic potion

Age-defying Athletes play, and, sometimes, they "pay" with an injury. But they always strive to get back in the game.

Participants in this research project report numerous fun, fitness, and friendship benefits from running around tennis courts, swinging golf clubs, crab walking pickleball games, propelling themselves through water, and jumping, sliding, skipping, tossing, twisting, and otherwise calling upon their body parts.

Benefits, yes. But every benefit carries a cost.

That's not surprising.

How many leaps have 70-year-old knees completed? No wonder they are as balky as teenagers.

And what about hips that have swiveled many, many times in the past 80 years? They shout, "No more twisting!" and tell their owners to go away.

Rotator cuffs are the multi-taskers of the upper body – tossing, catching, lifting, reaching. They're sick and tired of it and have gone on strike.

Backs? Was there a mention of backs that have held their owners up for 60, 70, 80, even 90 years? How are they doing?

Wrists, elbows, hamstrings, quads, groins, glutes, abdominals, even skin – select a favorite anatomical part and watch the injury expense tick up and up and up...

ADAP injury overview

Approximately 70% of over-age-50 Age-defying Athletes experienced harm in connection with their sport of choice.

Impairment occurred across genders and sport types. The only activities reporting no injury were yoga, ping-pong and softball. However, each was an N=1, so take that with a grain of salt.

To a person, however, the hurt individuals were committed to minimizing their sidelined time and to returning to their games as rapidly as possible. As one 76-year-old tennis player put it: "Rotator cuff surgery kept me out six months. Everybody wants to get over this sort of thing ASAP, and so did I."

The Masters Athletes research referenced earlier in this book found that their subjects feel they same way. They are keenly sensitive to the "use it or lose it" proposition and resist being forced back to the bench.

These researchers report, "In the words of the participants, they were strongly motivated by the concern that if they stopped being active through sport they will become 'old,' 'rusty,' 'age badly,' 'dependent on others,' or 'end up in [an aged care] home.'"[39]

In order not to feel old or rusty, some ADAPers will compensate for a "blacked out" sport with another activity.

Belinda, a tennis player, walked when a broken left elbow kept her away from the courts. In true Age-defying Athlete fashion, of course, Belinda eventually worked up to daily seven mile walks "to keep muscles tuned and also to maintain stamina"!

Age-defying Athlete injury specifics

In ADAP, the *biggest "cost"* paid for a benefit is a sport injury that (a) requires time off from the sport, and (b) necessitates professional intervention, such as from a physician, surgeon, physical therapist, massage therapist, or similar. Approximately 26% of all ADAP participants "paid" the largest "bill".

ADAP tennis players experienced the highest rate of "large bills" – almost half of those with an impairment fell into this category.

Nate, 73, for example, is an Age-defying tennis player who lost ten weeks for each of three ankle replacements.

A smaller percentage of ADAP golfers - 15% - forked over for large "hurt invoices" that necessitated time off plus professional care.

One pickleball player was debilitated enough to require time off and medical attention. So was one cyclist, Ruth, whose story is coming up later in this chapter.

The *second most expensive harm* is one that is serious enough for time off but does not require intervention. Another 17% of ADAP respondents have been "charged" this way.

Golfers were much more likely than tennis players to take time off from the links without professional care – 11 vs. three. None of the other athletes paid the time-off only price.

Third priciest for ADAP are conditions that are annoying, but require neither time off nor a professional look-see. Two tennis players and three golfers gutted it out this way, as did one each for pickleball, marathon, squash, triathlon, and cycling

Finally are *non-sport related circumstances* that block the athlete from participating - usually for months at a time. Four tennis players were impacted by cancer, as were three golfers.

An 88-year-old rower experienced a serious tumble down her home stairs and was hospitalized for three days; she was off the water for five weeks.

One tennis player developed a serious photo sensitivity and had to hang up her racquet for good at age 81.

The swimmer missed a couple of weeks for mole removal.

And several others lost time for other reasons such as work, travel, and caregiving.

Big picture stats

ADAP statistics run a bit counter to data from the National Safety Council (NSC).[40]

For example, ADAP tennis players were more prone to injury than ADAP golfers. However, in 2022, the NSC found that the rate of injury for golfers over age 65 was 41 per 100,000 population, whereas the number was 13 per 100,000 for racquet sports.

Additional NSC statistics:

- Swimming 23 per 100,000 for population 65+
- Softball 7 per 100,000 for population 65+

One ADAP pickleball player suffered challenges that caused her to stop her sport and seek medical attention. The NSC tracks no specific pickleball injuries, but the American Orthopedic Society for Sports Medicine[41] reports that in 2023, 19,000 pickleball-related injuries occurred in the US, with 29% of those in the lower body, and 33% in the upper body.

Most "expensive" injuries, as described by some ADAP participants

As noted above, these injuries require professional intervention plus a break from the sport.

Astrid

It's tough to be sidelined by injury from the one thing you do to stay active – especially if you are 88.

And especially if you have been tennis "royalty"...

To properly appreciate Astrid's tennis and injury story, it helps to remember the 70s – especially if you're in your 70s today.

Even if you're not in your 70s, you probably recall bell bottoms, hot pants, leisure suits...Stevie Wonder's "Superstition"... *Saturday Night Fever, Rocky,* and *Blazing Saddles.*

Nixon left the White House and Elvis left the planet.

Leading up to the 70s, students had perfected collegiate circadian rhythm: sleep until noon, dart off to afternoon classes, then invest endless hours debating, discussing, dissecting Life, Art, Sex, People, Philosophy, Blah, Blah, Blah.

Life, indeed! Before they knew it, those former students were living first jobs, and were jolted into a new sleep cycle: arise at 6AM, and then dart off to the gas station conga line to fill their tanks.

Insufficient gas (thanks, oil embargo) wasn't the only thing for which people awoke early.

To secure a court at a public tennis facility, players had to arrive in the wee hours and write their names on the clipboard affixed to the chain link fence surrounding the courts. (Cheat at this and you were instantly a racquet pariah. Who knows how they knew, but they knew.)

Courts were scarce enough to be fought over because America was not merely short on oil, it was long on tennis. A tennis frenzy, to be more precise.

Numerous factors drove this craze, the following two of particular interest to Astrid's tale:

In 1973, at the Houston Astrodome, Bobby Riggs and Billie Jean King played an exhibition match dubbed "The

Battle of the Sexes". It was watched by approximately 50 million people world-wide. Twenty-nine-year-old King bested Riggs, 55, in three sets.

Four years earlier, and to somewhat less than world-wide publicity, the Houston Racquet Club[42] (HRC) opened.

So what? Well, HRC is significant because this was the birthplace of Women's Professional Tennis in the US – and, arguably, the world.

In 1970, the "Original 9"[43] signed $1 contracts to play in the very first Virginia Slims tournament which was held at that Houston club – over the strenuous objection of the USTA.

The contracts were signed at the home of Gladys Heldman, an HRC member and founder and owner of *World Tennis* magazine.

Virginia Slims morphed into the Women's Tennis Association (WTA).

88-year-old Astrid, an Age-defying Athlete, was in the thick of it.

She and her second husband joined the new HRC even before its official Grand Opening. And that's how she started playing serious tennis.

Serious tennis at HRC involved serious training. "I took lessons from Jerry Evert, Chris' uncle."

He taught her to "watch them as they get ready to hit" – to look at the angle of an opponent's racquet face.

More lessons came from Owen Davidson and Manfred Joachim. Jimmy Parker also taught her. He was ranked the #1 US pro for years and focused on "moving the feet".

It wasn't just the hours spent learning the game. In the

spirit of the era she played and played and played: tennis three times a day, sometimes seven days a week. (Do the math.)

In something of an understatement, Astrid declares: "It was a very intense tennis period. It seemed that tennis was the only thing in the whole world."

Intense, indeed, with singles, doubles, mixed doubles with her husband, lots of competitions.

Spending so much time on the courts, she became quite skilled and was highly ranked as both a singles and doubles player. At one point, Astrid was USTA sectional champion and among the top 10 in the USA. In 1978, she was ranked seventh in Texas.

Eventually, Astrid earned one national singles ranking. Plus, she and her partner won a ladies national doubles tournament.

Astrid and her husband were quite the power couple, as well. In 1974 and 1976, the pair won the HRC club championship.

They didn't merely play the game, they lived it. Astrid and spouse had a house on a Houston street called Timberwild. "This street of only about ten houses," she recalls, "had five tennis courts – ours was in our front yard."

Timberwild was also the street where Gladys Heldman lived. As indicated earlier, Heldman was a major influence on the formation of women's tennis as a phenomenon. She and Billie Jean King had organized the women's pro tour in 1970 at HRC.

Astrid and Gladys became great friends. "She had a sign," Astrid remembers, "that 'tennis is the only sport where love is nothing.'"

Whether or not love is nothing or everything, by the late 1980s, Astrid fluctuated between nothing and everything tennis-wise. This continued into the 2000s.

Her tennis story circled back around by the 21st century: "I just went back [to tennis], and played sectionals and nationals on grass."

In 2019, she and her partner participated in national finals on clay courts in the 75-85 age track. Astrid was 83 at the time. "My partner and I," she believes, "would probably have won if we could have competed in the 85+ section."

Looking back on her superb life in tennis, Astrid notes, "I'm competitive and want to be accepted. I like being part of a group, whether I win or not."

She expands on this: "Having rank is less important than being part of a group at similar level. At the Houston Racquet Club, one would never invite a more highly ranked player to play. There were taboos about skill levels and one did not 'play up'."

"Tennis," Astrid continues, "is a great social sport...I'm a very social person."

Still competing in doubles twice a week, Astrid's goal is to "just keep playing."

That's especially meaningful in light of what happened a year ago to this woman who once was (and still is considered by some to be) a court elite. Even she couldn't escape an injury during a game.

"I fell and was concussed and out for six months. My therapy was to lie on a table as the tech turned me up and down in a sitting position. Then, as I lay there, I turned my head to relocate otoconia in my ears." Otoconia, Astrid adds, are "...hairs that attach to hearing crystals."

Astrid reports that she has completed eight rounds of therapy, but that "I still have some dizziness periodically so need to return again. Dehydration exacerbates this."

She has to serve underhanded now because the risk of dizziness prevents her from tilting her head up for the ball toss. (Nonetheless, word is that her serve is as un-returnable as ever.)

While she was recovering, Astrid affirms, "I missed not playing, not being part of a group. Scared to give tennis up because it's one way I do stay active."

Ruth

An ADAP cyclist also incurred a "highest pricetag" due to a riding mishap. This perhaps may not be surprising, as the NSC cites bicycle injuries as relatively high, with a 65 and older rate of 95 per 100,000 population.[44]

It all began when Ruth, 65, and her husband decided to start cycling to help them prepare for a hundred mile hike through the Swiss, French, and Italian Alps in the summertime. They targeted 10 to 12 miles hiked per day for 10 to 12 days. Their schedule also included allowance for one rest day.

Bicycling, Ruth explains, was "...completely a sideline thing for hiking. I wanted to get my legs stronger for longer, harder hikes."

And, in point of fact, hiking itself was a "sideline thing".

"Eleven years ago, our daughter wanted two puppies. One of them was very high energy, so my husband and I started hiking around town to wear them out. Then we started going to different places and wanted to go farther away for hikes a few years later."

That first year, they ventured as far afield as Glacier National Park, Montana. "We worked up to 42 miles a week. We saw amazing things we couldn't see from a car."

Ruth continues, "We were planning to see Grand Teton that summer, and planned to go to the gym to increase fitness. We thought that rather than drive to the club, 'Let's bicycle [there] for extra workout.'"

They began by riding regular bicycles through their hilly neighborhood. But, she admits, "that was hard…"

Ruth adds that "My biggest fear back then was being run over by a car. I didn't expect to fall. But I don't want to let fear keep me back."

Eventually, they purchased ebikes to facilitate their rides.

"We looked at ebikes at an electric bike store," Ruth relates. "We tried them out, liked them, but [the bike shop] had no way of delivering them to us. So, we explored online and found Upway Bikes.[45] We bought two Gazelles. [They were] shipped with a 14 day guarantee. Bicycles were completely assembled, except for pedals."

Ruth recounts that as a young girl, on her banana bike, "I rode downhill too fast, the bike started shaking and I went splat on a gravel road."

More than half a century later, she relived this experience.

In June last year – as they were gearing up for their Grand Teton National Park trip - Ruth recalls, "I was going downhill toward spin class, and stopped quickly and toppled over, with the bicycle on my knee. I couldn't get up, then my husband helped me."

At that point, she attempted to pedal, but was unable to do so. Her husband "advised me to just use the electronic assist to get home – without pedaling. I got home, but within two hours, I couldn't walk."

The couple eventually made the trip to Grand Teton. "I did ten miles wearing a knee brace, on a cortisone shot, but the shot wore off after that."

The following September, Ruth had knee surgery, followed by a couple months of twice-weekly physical therapy.

Before that surgical procedure, she admits, "I had gotten back [after the initial injury] way too soon and didn't think I could stop the bicycle because I had no stable leg then. After surgery, my leg was stable."

Ever mindful of regaining her leg strength following these various difficulties, Ruth reports that "I tried spin class last Friday for 50 minutes with zero resistance, but even that was too long."

But, consistent with other ADAP interviewees, she is focused on getting back on the bike and minimizing additional lost time. Nowadays, she is up to one or two rides each week.

Despite her banana bike tumble, Ruth confesses to being surprised by her fall. "We try and research everything, and chance of injury was an area where I hadn't thoroughly researched."

Still, she is an ebike fan. They are "great bikes, but I have to be careful. Great for older people. Even though I have been injured, I can pedal hard or not."

All in all, however, cycling has benefitted her. "I have stronger legs. I wouldn't have picked [cycling] up just to pick it up.

"Everything is based on hiking. I want to get my legs stronger. If I am more confident, I will bike more, go longer distances."

Second most "expensive" injuries, as described by some ADAP participants

These are the harms requiring time off, but that do not require professional intervention.

Henry

Henry didn't play any sports growing up until he was a high school exchange student in Portugal.

"I was living with a Portuguese family whose children were sports nuts," he relates. "I didn't speak Portuguese, so classes were difficult for me. I had nothing else to do, so tagged along with them and started playing hockey, soccer, a form of indoor handball."

In 1970, when he was 23, he began participating in tennis, mostly because his girlfriend at the time had just accepted a job with a brand new tennis center. "No one was using the courts yet, so they encouraged staff to play and I took it up."

Over the years – after hitting a ball over the fence around

a rooftop court on a five story building – he took lots and lots of lessons.

Recently, Henry experienced his first groin pull while on the courts. "I had to stop playing immediately. I went home and used heat, cold, pressure, and it was gone in three days."

There were also racquet-related physical challenges in the past. "I had tennis elbow on and off for five or six years," this 77-year-old tennis player relates. "...and then I finally discovered a light pressure bandage would do the trick."

He didn't enjoy quite such an easy time with other injuries, however. "I developed sciatica from driving a manual Mustang and was out [from tennis] six weeks."

To ease the pain, he says that he "...slid my butt over a hard roller and that pressed on the nerve and that helped."

Hudson

An elbow challenge also reared up for Hudson, who is a fairly recent convert to the golf links, having launched into the game about a year ago.

This embrace of golf was probably one of those epiphanies occurring after a major life event, because Hudson joined a golf club the day after being released from the hospital for a heart condition.

Then, he says, "I tweaked an elbow tendon and was out one and a half months. I felt pretty good, and had no expectations of playing well, and that's how I bounced back."

Third most "expensive" injury, as described by some ADAP participants

Annoying, yes, but these injuries demand neither intervention nor time off.

Asami

"A couple of years ago, I dove for a [pickleball] ball just as it came over the net. Didn't get ball back, but I broke my finger and had a huge knot on my head for days. I didn't stop playing, however!"

Asami, 77, began the sport "five or six years ago".

The reason she started the game is that "One year, our Vermont son sent a pickleball set to our [northern] summer cabin and we set it up in the driveway. Driveway couldn't completely accommodate pickleball boundaries, so our grandson was charged with figuring out how to make it 10% smaller."

Once the family had the revised dimensions, they marked them off with chalk. Unfortunately, "After a rain, however, chalk marks would vanish, so the next summer, we painted lines for the court."

Further adjustment still required! Asami notes that "... when playing, we have to move the net from the lawn to the driveway, and close the garage door."

Par for the course for a woman who has played tennis for more than 50 years, and describes her family as "athletic".

"All this time, we mostly play on the driveway 'court',

but also on a court at the community center and at our club."

When she played at the club, it was her first time on a regulation pickleball court. "The service court appeared to be a long way away," Asami remarks.

Whether or not related to this perception, nowadays Asami is having "...a hard time serving the ball. Thought about practicing on driveway. Had a serve for awhile, but then it went away just like [serve disappears] in tennis."

Also some not surprising advice, given her injury: "Don't ever run after a ball, just let it go. Maybe the player will believe he or she can get to the ball due to the smaller court," cautions Asami. Since it's a competitive environment, it's tempting to run. But she repeats: "Don't run for balls."

All in all, she summarizes, "I get a little discouraged if I cannot perform basics [such as the serve]. But like with golf, you either quit or you improve And I'm going to improve."

Blossom

While not nearly as dramatic as Asami's impairment, Blossom, 58, reports that she has "not really" had any injuries, nor taken any time off from playing squash.

After considering a moment, however, she adds, "I have had some plantar fasciitis, but it's not a major thing."

Fourth most "expensive" injury, as described by some ADAP participants

These are non-sports circumstances that necessitated time off. And in the case of the seven ADAP cancer patients, significant medical intervention was also required.

Mildred

Mildred, who perfected her backhand through mirroring that of Steffi Graff (Chapter 4), can look back on more than 50 years of playing tennis.

Like numerous other ADAP respondents, she had little formal childhood experience with any sport. "...Dance as kid – ballet, tap, jazz. In college, I only took required [physical education] courses."

She describes how, in her 20s, she began the game of tennis: "Girlfriends at work were starting a foursome and asked if I wanted in. As a kid, when bored, I had hit balls on side of house, which helped hand-eye coordination..."

Scheduling play was difficult because it required aligning the schedules of four women in the midst of their careers.

Which may be why they took no lessons at the beginning. "No one was serious, we were just horsing around. However," Mildred adds, "as [our] interest grew, we took lessons and formed a USTA league team."

Over the decades, Mildred and her teams achieved regional and national rankings.

Her upward trajectory came to a halt about four years

ago. "Breast cancer was diagnosed in May 2020 and I had to back off about six months."

During that period, she relates, "I would hit a bit, but couldn't play serious game. Biggest challenge coming back was mobility and strength in my left arm."

Because her pre-cancer backhand style had been two-handed, Mildred took drills to learn to hit one-handed again.

But it paid an unexpected dividend. "In the process, I learned to slice, which I had never had."

She affirms, "I bounced back mostly by taking time to recover."

If there is a silver lining to Mildred's story, it's that her treatment "...happened during COVID, so I didn't miss much of [league] season."

In reminiscing about the decades of sport experiences, she says that "For me, biggest thing [in tennis] is the social aspect. Most of the people I am close with I have met through tennis or Jazzercize® [which she taught for many years]. Challenge is trying to be better at it and continue to try to win."

Estrella

Golfer Estrella, 59, should have followed the 1950s refrigerator magnet wisdom that "Housework won't kill you, but why take a chance?"

Laundry was the culprit for Estrella. She injured her wrist pulling down a bottle of detergent in her utility room.

"Turns out to have been a really bad sprain, so I backed

off two-and-a-half weeks, but then played a tournament last week and wrist turned bad afterward," she explains. "So, very frustrated and concerned because I'm worried about my game."

Wilton

Wilton is a 64-year-old golfer who has plied the links for over 40 years.

Similar to Mildred's reason for deciding to start a sport, he began the game because "Guys at work played and asked me to join them."

Growing up, he participated in plenty of athletics. "...I was pretty good at sports, making the varsity basketball team as a sophomore at a large high school – more than 750 grads. I had grown up around sports, so knew I would continue with athletic pursuits."

His initial golf lesson, however, wasn't until he was 32, after attempting the game for ten years. "First lesson from Samantha was in 1992."

Reflecting both his athletic upbringing as well as the "fit" with an instructor, Wilton eventually excelled at the game: "From 1992 to 1996, I went to a seven handicap. Samantha had to make me think differently."

Wilton describes the game as benefitting him several ways: "Health. Friends. Because I can no longer play basketball, due to various joint issues, golf keeps me more active than I might be otherwise."

He categorizes golf as "... my outlet to be competitive.

During a tournament, my Fitbit® records four-and-a-half hours of cardio, so competitive tournaments elevate my heart rate."

A student of the game, Wilton attempts to keep up practice and lessons in the midst of a demanding job: "Once a week in spring and summer, I go to the driving range to practice. Wish I could take more lessons, and will try to do two a month during peak season. Play with Samantha on Sundays, so she can comment on little things which is kind of a mini lesson."

"I have a bad back, so I stretch twice a day," Wilton adds.

Ironically, despite this pre-existing condition, Wilton's injury apparently didn't involve his back.

He is an avid oenophile as well as golfer. Unfortunately, Wilton's injury brought these two interests together.

"There was no medical intervention but I injured my left shoulder moving wine boxes and took four to six weeks off....Somehow - I don't know how – I also injured my right shoulder and took a couple of weeks off."

He attributes his recess from the links to "Old age – takes longer to heal."

Reynaldo, Hans, Murten, Blair, Leon, Lawton, Crawford

Several Age-defying Athletes such as Reynaldo, the "sixty-something" marathoner, and 60-year-old bicyclist Hans, have missed competition due to work demands.

Murten, the 59-year-old golfer, took a break from the game to care for her seriously ill Mother.

Several golfers declare a hiatus when summer heat is oppressive.

Blair 62, misses some tennis "...due to travel, but I just slid back in [upon return]. Sometimes when we travel, I take a lesson or join a drill wherever we are."

Golfer Leon, 80, took a recess due to kidney stone surgery.

Lawton, 76, reports that he has endured "...a mysterious pulmonary problem for over a year. Somewhat better, but still a daily challenge."

Crawford, 66, lost about three months from tennis about a year and a half ago. "I broke my ankle when stepping out of my daughter's car at a soccer field. Stepped into a gap alongside the curb and went over with my body weight."

The bone was not dislocated, this player notes, "So I wore a walking cast for a few weeks."

McGregor

86-year-old McGregor talks about an injury that impacted his golf game: "Four years ago, I hurt my right shoulder lifting weights."

Despite this, he remarks, "I played with a bad shoulder for two years...[My] daughter talked me into shoulder replacement surgery in Manchester, New Hampshire, where she lived."

Due to the procedure, his daughter took care of him and his wife for the period surrounding the surgery.

Unfortunately, "It took another two years before I was

pain free. I went through several rehabs: five months in New Hampshire, another six months in my home state, plus three more months in New Hampshire."

Emerging from rehab, he chipped for a few months.

"Even after one year post surgery," he adds, "there were restrictions. Only in the last couple of years have I felt I could get the club around my shoulder, up to the top of my swing."

They play, they pay – but they renew themselves

Almost all human endeavor requires some sort of trade-off, some balance of play and payment, of cost and benefit.

And so it is for Age-defying Athletes. They recognize that they will have to trade off time, energy, money, and more for their sports. That's part of the risk of stepping "out there" for a game.

But the benefits outweigh the costs for the ADAP community. They are renewed by that elixir which provides friendship, fun, fitness, fresh air, mental sharpness, and more.

That's why they are always anxious to minimize time away and maximize time back. They need the revitalization that their games deliver.

Chapter 9
Not Fifty, but still Nifty

Lowering the drinking age

The 92 Age-defying Athletes whose stories swing, run, jump, glide, leap, and otherwise vibrate through these pages are all over 50 years old. (They are astonishing, yes?)

However, as part of the research for this book, five more athletes were interviewed, and they all had lived for less than a half century.

Was relative youth a significant factor in the behavior of the under-50 crowd vs. the group 50 and older?

Not significant, no.

The Nifties' youth seemed to seriously differentiate them mainly in one area: no serious injury. Only one of the five experienced any injury requiring time off, and hers was merely a self-exile without professional intervention.

The other factor in which there was a bit of difference between the two age cohorts was in experience level. All five Nifties were Sports Virgins, whereas that category only applied to a segment of the older athletes.

Other than these variables, the youngsters' experiences have paralleled those of the more senior population. Apparently the "lower drinking age" enabled these men and women to also take advantage of the elixir of sport.

Snapshot of the five Nifties:

Sport	Males	Females	Average age (per sport)	Number of interviewees
Tennis	0	2	44	2
Golf	1	0	40	1
Pickleball	1	1	43	2
Subtotals	2	3		5

• Overall average age is 43, with a range of 38 to 47
• Before beginning their sport, they had been inactive for about 14 years. The years of inactivity range is not telling, however, as one man and one woman reported zero years of inactivity; but another women hadn't done anything "sports-wise" for 30 years.
• Nifties took up their game when they were almost 40 years old.
• The men grew up playing sports, but only one of the women did.
• One of the men expected to be (and was) an athlete as an adult; the other four had had no athlete dreams nor fulfillment.
• They participate roughly twice a week, with the two tennis players competing as frequently as four times weekly.

Why did they begin?

The older cohort of Age-defying Athletes decided to play for a fairly broad array of reasons – fitness, friendship, family, fun, something to do in retirement, and more.

A somewhat different decision dynamic affected the under-50 group. While their resolve to play a game rested on five distinct stories, their tales had lots of similar components.

The pickleball player, Arne, 38, heard of pickup pickleball from his neighbor: "It seemed an easy thing to try."

Encouragement from others also influenced Walter, who is 40 and explains that when he retired from an athletic career four years ago, he decided to buckle down and play golf.

"A few [professional athletes] I know would invite me to sometimes play in tournaments, but golf sucks if you don't play well," notes Walter, who added, "After I retired in 2019, at age 36, I decided I had the time, so let me just do it."

For the women, COVID played a part in their decisions for both tennis and pickleball.

"COVID hit and I wanted to be outside and exercising," states Nelli, 43, "so tennis checked a lot of boxes. Three other girls wanted to play, too, so we went to a court in our neighborhood and one of them convinced a pro to meet us there. He gave us lessons for about six months."

Additionally, she says, "I was at a time in my life when my kids were beginning to be independent. I wanted something just for me. Tennis was something I could schedule in two hour blocks, so it was convenient."

Similarly, the outdoors during COVID influenced Thelma, 45.

"I am a certified yoga instructor. My goal had been to quit my [professional] job to conduct yoga retreats," she explains. "I did quit [my job] in 2019 and took tennis lessons as a lead up to retirement. This accelerated during COVID, as I was uncomfortable inside with yoga, and there wasn't a lot of outside yoga available."

Rebeka, 47, echoes much of this: "During COVID, we looked for something to do. Previously I had gone to movies every weekend with girlfriends, but movies were out so I started researching pickleball."

How did they prepare?

As with the Age-defying Athlete over-50 segment, this younger cohort was split between lesson-takers and do-it-yourselfers.

All the female players took lessons.

"I found a private instructor who teaches [pickleball] at a court in an apartment complex," reports Rebeka. "He also teaches tennis there. Took group lessons with [my] other three friends – basics, scoring, paddles. Still play with him observing, or sometimes he will fill in as a participant."

"I took basic group [tennis] lessons," notes Thelma.

For Nelli, tennis preparation meant: "I took lots of drills."

The men did it themselves, at least at first.

"Tried it for myself at first, because I can pick up just about any sport," explains Walter. "But my hand-eye coordination and golf technique were humbling. So, after a few months of beating the grass, I took lessons."

"Just went out," recalls Arne, "...borrowed a paddle."

What was the most difficult aspect of starting?

"Difficulty was that from football," where Walter had had a successful career, "a lot doesn't carry over. Tense for football, fluid in golf.

"Mental, anger in football, go harder and be more aggressive."

But that is incompatible with golf. "Going harder won't work," he declares.

Additionally, Walter describes other contrasts between the links and the gridiron: "I'm around golf people and get tips. In sports [such as football], not a lot of guidance, just do what you do. But in golf everyone helps. I can tell others how to hit, even."

Golf is less forgiving than football, too. "Difficult doing the same thing, [with] consistency. To take back [golf] swing, and do it the same way, hit the ball in the center of the face every time. As much as an inch or centimeter off, you're off. In football, I can compensate."

Thelma experienced a different kind of challenge at the beginning. "There was the anxiety about spending money when I was no longer working."

But, she continues, "Tennis is a hobby, something to

get out of the regularity of my life. Not difficult to start. I wanted stress relief through competition."

Competition had a different impact on Nelli when she was starting: "Difficulty comparing myself to other players and seeing how they progressed when I didn't think I was. Hard to watch."

For Rebeka, the start-up challenge centered on her playing partners. "I was worried my friends wouldn't like [pickleball] and then I wouldn't have anyone to play with."

She lives in a major metropolitan area whose traffic congestion is so thick, residents rarely venture much beyond perhaps a five mile radius of home. Thus, pickleball courts and partners can be scarce – and treasured.

What has the playing experience been like?

Arne observes "Wide range of people from beginner to tournament calibre participate [in pickleball]. Competitive but informal."

Echoing a common description of pickleball, he adds that the game is "...just mainly fun."

Rebeka is surprised by the assortment of people who play the sport: "Doesn't matter age, athleticism, body type, anyone can excel at pickleball. There's not a pickleball 'type'. Really everyone is nice and friendly, all about being in good company and having fun."

Rebeka is enthusiastic about her sport. "I am addicted. I

get the hype around the game. When I am able to retire, I'd like to become a senior pro pickleball player!"

She also "...follows some newsletters on social media."

Nelli is similarly energized. "Absolutely love tennis," she exclaims. "I play almost every day. Main form of exercise, local league and two USTA teams."

A thought-provoking cloud blocks her sunny perspective, however.

"As I have reached more advanced levels with more competition," explains Nelli, "I miss my happy-go-lucky tennis. Advancing rapidly, as I have, is very satisfying, but there is more player drama [within teams at higher levels] such as people already jumping from one team to another for next season. There's a price to play at these more advanced levels."

Thelma is enthralled with the court game. "I love it. It's fun. I have met lovely people. Gives me a sense of purpose – 'OK, this is what I'm doing.'"

Many over-50 ADAP participants saw sports as a way to integrate into a new community. Along these lines, Thelma adds a comment about how relocating to a new town influenced her decision to play tennis. But her selection came with a twist: "I'm not sure I would have been into tennis as much if we hadn't moved here. Part of overall move gestalt."

Walter's experience? "Golf is a sport where quality time is a value – with friends, for business. Big time quality time," he claims.

In fact, now he has reached a level of links competence in which playing doesn't claim all his attention anymore. "Nowadays, golf is no longer a distraction to being with friends or business acquaintances. I cannot say I've conquered golf. I've arrived somewhere."

Of course, there's always that consistency thing. "But the next day, I've not arrived. There are so many aspects of this game to conquer."

How have these Nifties benefitted from playing?

"Physical, social, aggression and competitiveness outlet," admits Rebeka. "It's a great conversation piece. I took new job a month ago. People either want to try pickleball or, if it's a tennis person, I always say, 'You don't like me'. Breaks the ice."

She adds, "Even if someone is non-athletic, they should try it just once to see what it's like. I've tried lots of things, like hatchet throwing."

Walter describes what golf has done for him: "Made me more patient. Patience is not a virtue in football, but it is in golf. Take your time. Next shot most important one."

He has also made a discovery about himself: "I can do anything I put my mind to. I can hit a straight tee shot. Well on my journey."

Advantages for Thelma are: "I'm more active, meeting people, have a sense of purpose."

She also has had an unusual self-discovery: "I wanted something I wouldn't be good at. The idea of sporty vs. intellectual. Let's have some fun. I knew I would have to work at it."

Nelli says that tennis is "definitely fantastic fitness and health thing for me. Keeps me young, keeps me moving."

Something she's discovered from playing is that "I can do hard, scary things. Given me confidence."

For Arne, camaraderie is a benefit he has received from playing pickleball. He states that, "Seeing improvement adds to my enjoyment." But Arne admits that "I definitely could improve if I would pay more attention."

Surprises

As far as eye-openers from their games, two of the women have been surprised that they perform as well as they do.

Nelli explains: "For me, the most surprising [thing about tennis] has been how good I was able to be in a short period of time without any athletic background."

And Thelma opines, "I don't suck as much as I thought I would. I win some and that surprises me."

Walter, the retired professional athlete, had the opposite emotional response – at least initially. He explains that "When just starting, I didn't want to play with anyone I knew because I feared embarrassing myself. Now, it's OK to lose balls. And if I play with an eight or 10 handicapper who hits a bad shot, I tell myself that looks just like my shots. It's always about the next shot."

"Surprise is how quickly this has been popularized nationwide," says Arne of pickleball.

Goals

Perhaps pickleball's popularity is one reason Arne's goal is "... to continue to play. I would like to find other opportunities than pickup and have thought about structured tournament play."

Thelma also takes the long perspective regarding tennis goals: "I would like to still play when I'm 90. Want to stay active, fit, outdoors. I also like being on a team."

Nelli, hearkening back to her comment about losing some of the happy-go-lucky sense of tennis as she climbed the expertise ladder, includes this in her goal: "Weighing where I want to sit with tennis. Trade off being strong player vs. camaraderie. Enjoyment vs. being good." (A similar tradeoff was called out by Juanita, the golfer, in Chapter 3.)

Rebeka's objective? She is a pragmatist: "I like to win, but this experience isn't about winning. Love to play at least one more time a week if my work schedule permits. Would also love to enter a tournament."

Walter's goal? He is also practical, commenting, "I want to play golf at least once a week, 18 holes. Sometimes twice a week."

Motivation

All five express lots of motivation to participate in their games.

As a competitive person, Walter says he stays motivated by "...just [going] out and playing...I don't want to waste time."

Motivation for Thelma means "I don't know how not to be motivated."

Nelli's conundrum of "fun" vs. "good" shapes her motivation to play: "I know there's a light at the end of the tunnel. I need to do a better job of figuring out what that looks like."

"Motivation is not an issue – playing is an excuse to have an opportunity to compete," summarizes Arne.

Similarly for Rebeka: "Motivation is not hard. We play Saturday mornings and always confirm for the next week. If someone cannot make it, I may join an earlier class and rotate through different combinations."

Injury

Four of the five experienced no injury requiring time off or professional intervention. Maybe youth captures the point in this realm?

Thelma was the only one to lay low for awhile, following a problem with a joint: "I did hurt my wrist playing tennis and waited it out for a couple of weeks. I was a little worried because a new season was about to begin, but no long term effects."

The others have had assorted aches and pains.

"Right wrist injured when I hit the ground attempting a shot," Walter reports. "But I didn't lose any time."

"I strained a calf muscle going for a shot," states Rebeka, who emphasizes that she got the shot anyway.

Another time, she was "...beaned in the jaw by the ball

and it temporarily dislocated. But nothing serious and I never took time off."

Arne still works, and his job can be a deterrent to participating in pickleball. "My work travel schedule sometimes keeps me from playing. Knock on wood, no injuries."

Family sometimes prevents Nelli from being on the court. "No injuries. Pretty lucky. Every once in a while, have a kiddo thing, such as a sick kid."

What about practicing their sports?

Thelma, Walter, and Nelli all report some effort at regular practice.

Nelli explains, "I don't do a lot off court, but have started Jazzercise and stretching. Drills with teams and separate weekly lesson in which I work on a variety of things."

Thelma also participates in tennis drills. "I work out with weights, but that's more for general fitness. Team drills, other drills."

"Definitely make time sporadically for range," Walter reports. He's also "planning to resume lessons."

Arne does not practice, nor does Rebeka. But she confirms that she tries to stretch before leaving to play.

In conclusion...

Except for injury and being Sports Virgins, the Nifties are strikingly similar to their older cohorts.

One conclusion is that men and women of all ages need renewal – it's not just a phenomenon of creaky Geezers.

Another conclusion is that this under-50 sample is ahead of the curve with respect to starting a sport. Certainly, plenty in the older pool began playing when they were in their late 30s-late 40s. However, lots of ADAPers didn't jump into a game until they were post-retirement, or at least in their 60s. Many of these lamented that they wish they had taken up a sport when they were younger.

All in all, it's a very, very good thing that the drinking age has been lowered.

Chapter 10
WIIFY?

Now it's your turn to brew some magic

What's in It for You?

WIIFY? is the most important question of all.

Throughout this book, Age-defying Athletes have hopped, flipped, and skipped toward renewal. Whether through physical re-invigoration, mental rejuvenation, the joy of camaraderie, or simply being "out there" where they breathe fresh air and wander in the great outdoors, ADAPers are getting better even as they are growing older.

"Growing older". That Dark Age when all growth, renewal, happiness, health, and fun shut down. Forever.

Forget that and bring on the self-refreshment! That's absolutely within your grasp.

To assist you, here are some of the key ideas you can take from this volume to encourage and maintain your own self-rejuvenation campaign.

They are organized to coincide with the main chapters of *The Elixir of Sport*.

Deciding

I have read about self-renewal in this book, but am not convinced I want to try a sport at this stage of my life.

Fair enough. Athletics may not be for everyone. But you would be challenged to identify a more <u>reliable</u> means of adding fun, fitness, and friendship to your existence.

Consider the ways that Age-defying Athletes decided to start (or return to or continue) playing:

- Urged by a spouse
- Saw people playing and were curious
- Read a book about a game
- Moved to a new community and wanted to meet people
- Felt like a slug and sought to become less slug-ly
- Filled a gap for something to do in the summertime
- Shamed by work colleagues into going along
- Wanted to find an activity to do in retirement

Do any of these apply to you?

Remember that it's not just ADAP that has identified fun, fitness, and friendship as goals that older adults pursue through playing sports. Two other sources reinforce this phenomenon.

What Retirees Want

Ken Dychtwald and Robert Morison, in their book *What Retirees Want*[46] (cited in Chapter 1) report that

"Staying healthy/improving health" topped the list of retiree leisure priorities, with 83% of respondents selecting it. Relaxing (72%), family connections (58%), fun (57%), and friendships/social connections (56%) rounded out the top five.[47]

Now that Baby Boomers have retired, the authors estimate, they globally have a whopping 50 trillion hours of leisure[48] to spend on those activities.

Even more important for self-renewal, Boomers intend to spend it differently than did their parents. "I want to keep growing and trying new things. I don't want to be as old as my parents were when they were this age,"[49] one retiree told Dychtwald and Morison.

For all those retirement hours headed your way, ask yourself:

- *Does my retirement differ from that of my parents?*
- *Is my vision about what retirees do a bit out-of-date, a tad too stereotype-laden?*
- *Is it genuinely mine?*

A good initial step toward self-renewal is to create a retirement that is uniquely yours, and that satisfies the criteria Dychtwald and Morison mention: health, socialization, family, fun, and relaxation.

You would do worse than playing sports – especially remembering that you need not play well!

Transamerica Center study

The Transamerica Center study (Chapter 1) quantified the need for ways to fill those leisure hours:

About 21% of retirees[50] – or 10 million individuals – worry that they will not find meaningful ways to spend their time. In fact, only about 40%[51] of them report pursuing hobbies.

Most retirees are upbeat. But some of them feel unmotivated and overwhelmed (26%) and are anxious and depressed (24%). 18% worry about "feeling isolated and alone".52

Pre-retirees aged 50+ tell a similar tale: 18% worry about finding meaningful ways to spend time; 31% are unmotivated and overwhelmed.[53]

People are looking for revitalization. They desire a new lease on life – especially once retirement has evaporated the structure they had while working (no matter how much or how little they enjoyed their jobs!).

It's just coffee

As you consider whether or not to start a sport, remember, "It's just coffee." You're not marrying a sport at the get-go. You're not even going steady yet!

Sample one or more athletic pastimes and decide whether that "special sauce" is there for you. If not, move on to something else, perhaps with the encouragement of a spousal unit or friend.

How to think about a sport for you

If you are intrigued by the possibility of revitalization, but haven't a clue about what sport to try, here are a few questions to ponder:

Solo or group?

- If you are more of an introvert, a solo sport such as swimming, cycling, marathoning, or triathloning may be the best fit. You can take things at your own pace, and the main competitor is yourself.
- More of an extrovert? Racquet sports, team games such as softball or soccer should be at the top of your list.
- Multi-faceted personality? Plenty of solo sports can be enjoyed in a group (think of Masters Swim teams, for example), and some team games may also be reduced to individual play. Rowing, for instance, can be performed by one to eight. And where does golf fit? It traverses the introvert-to-extrovert boundaries.

Fitness requirements?

You want to become fitter, but it takes a certain baseline level of fitness to get there.

The following distinctions are general guidelines, as any sport can be performed more or less vigorously.

<u>More fitness needed</u>
• Endurance sports such as running marathons and competing in triathlons will require solid levels of fitness.
• There's a lot of running in tennis and squash, too.
• You can master these with sufficient training, but it's not a good idea to just unfold from a sofa and launch an endurance athletic career.

<u>Less fitness needed</u>
• Pickleball is popular with older adults for a variety of reasons, one of which is that it can be played at a leisurely pace.
• Numerous readers will protest this, but softball involves a lot of standing around with bursts of action, so may be fitness intense or not.
• Golf demands good rotational coordination and the ability to swing clubs, but played from a golf cart, can be managed with less aerobic investment.
• And many feel that swimming is Zen.
• Cycling isn't just about screaming downhill, but can easily be performed in a gentle fashion – especially on an electric assist bike.
• And while yoga can be quite demanding, it is also meditative.

Expense?

Equipment, lessons, and memberships can be a small or large investment.

On the equipment side, there will always be a range of prices from tiny to eye-poppingly enormous. Used, borrowed or rented items can deliver big savings.

Regarding lessons, group training will typically be less costly per attendee than one-to-one coaching. Even better, "Friends & Family" training may be free – except for the shared memory of how bad you were when you began (just kidding...).

And on the membership side, rely on free public facilities – especially if conveniently available.

More costly new equipment
- A set of golf clubs can easily run into four figures.
- Likewise for a sizzling bicycle for triathlons or road racing. "Tris" also call for expensive wet suits.
- Top end tennis and squash racquets can cost several hundred dollars.

Less costly new equipment
- Pickleball paddles generally are priced from $70-150.
- A good quality swimsuit, goggles, and cap probably will set the swimmer back about $100-150.
- A top notch pair of running shoes goes for $100-200 these days. (But if you are a marathoner or "tri," expect to go through several pair annually.)
- A yoga mat can be purchased for less than $100.

Infrastructure?

How much trouble will it be to pursue your sport? For example, if you're crazy about the links, are you crazy enough to drive an hour each way to play? And if tennis is your passion, can you find enough players for regular games? Rowing requires water, and swimming, a pool – are these available?

It is worth your time to assess whether or not your sport of choice will choose you.

Support system?

Any fine and upstanding adult is certainly capable of commencing an athletic career on his or her lonesome. But it can be easier if some sort of support system exists.

Do you have a spouse who is already ga-ga for a sport? This can ease your introduction to that particular game.

But, on the other hand, a ga-ga spouse may be a turn-off for that particular athletic selection.

Kids can provide support. Asami was propelled into pickleball when her son sent a set including net, paddles, balls, and instructions to the family's summer cabin.

Friends are good guides to the world of athletics. They have experience in the local environment and can provide tips on pros and facilities to avoid and those to choose. Plus, a shared game is a great way to enrich those bonds of camaraderie.

As you consider whether or not to pursue a game, these

are just some of the variables that can shape a positive or negative sporting experience. What others come to mind?

Preparing

Even if I wanted to give it a try, I haven't a clue how to begin.

Perhaps, like some Age-defying Athletes, you never expected to play a game in later life. Your interest could have evolved, however, and now you are curious to see what it might be like to follow a little white ball down a big green parkway or scamper after a bouncing yellow one on a carpet of blue.

It is an ADAP principle that each person carries a seed of athleticism. The question is: what's the mystery mix to encourage that seed to bloom?

In other words, How to prepare? How to prepare?

Books

Some Age-defying Athletes began by reading a book.

Reynaldo, the proud father marathoner, read Jeff Galloway's *Run Walk Run* and used that as a basis for training.

Winston and Cora launched their competitive "career" with *Slow, Fat Triathlete*.

(Details on both in Chapter 11.)

The helpful thing about books is that you can sample several sports before deciding to try one. There are starter volumes on tennis, golf, pickleball, swimming, running, bicycling, triathlons, and much more. If you check a couple out from the library (in person or online), you don't even have to fork over your hard-earned cash.

Observation

Maybe "first, observe" is your preferred approach to trying something new. The web, of course, provides gazillions of YouTube videos of every sport imaginable – as well as some you probably never imagined.

If you would rather observe in 3D, real time, check out your community's recreational sports facilities. Maybe the men's over-50 softball league is playing and you can catch a few innings. Or, visit a rec center and ask to take a look at their pool or ping-pong area or pickleball courts (or all three!).

Try it

After observing, you may simply decide to give it a try. Plenty of Age-defying Athletes took up their sport without formal instruction; they just leaped out and started playing.

If this sounds like you, and, for instance, the links are calling, consider borrowing or renting golf clubs and spending time experimenting at a driving range.

Pickleball is new and wide open, so lots of would-be dinkers simply show up to public courts for open play and swing. Someone may loan you a paddle or you can inquire about renting one.

Learn it

In contrast, perhaps you value instruction and want to learn a sport the right way right from the start. Across the USA, almost every game has thousands of group clinics and individual classes. For example, if tennis intrigues you, check out the USTA website for ideas. (Details in next chapter.)

Coaching

Recognize that throughout the skill spectrum – that is, for rookies, competents, and experts – coaching can deliver an important contribution. The newbies simply need to learn what to do, while the experts want to learn to do it better.

Satisfying this instructional demand is a large supply of professionals at tennis clubs, golf courses, pickleball facilities, swimming pools, rowing clubs, fitness centers, and more.

Two examples quantify the coach "supply" out there:

According to the Tennis Industry Association, the US has approximately 15,000 tennis facilities.[54]

The National Golf Foundation says that in 2020, the US

had about 16,100 courses at 14,100 facilities. 75% of these are open to the public.[55]

The decision to lesson or not to lesson depends on a multitude of factors: time, facility availability, motivation (i.e., how arduous will this learning task be, and what are you willing to sacrifice to meet the demands?), cost, and more.

You also must be honest with yourself about the long-term commitment to the sport – is this potentially a lifelong pursuit, or a momentary curiosity?

Finally, what is your current skill level?

There is no right or wrong answer about coaching and lessons here.

However, in general, if you are a <u>Sports Virgin</u> who is motivated to stick with a sport for more than one season, experiment with a lesson. Don't sign up for a year's worth of them (!). And try to borrow equipment rather than investing in whatever the game demands.

In other words, ease in slowly. (It's just coffee, remember?)

Keep in mind, too, that the first instructor or class you take may not be your cup of tea (mixing beverage metaphors here). Don't let an unsatisfactory lesson turn you off to the sport. Go elsewhere, and be clear about what you seek from a pro.

<u>Prodigals</u> and <u>Continuers</u> may also want to consider similar advice.

If, as a Prodigal, you are stepping back into a game you enjoyed more than a decade ago, go out and "just do it," but keep in mind that a coach may help you address some of the …er…rustier parts of your play.

Are you a Continuer? You, too, could periodically benefit from having your game refreshed. Maybe you don't think instruction could help, or perhaps you feel you are doing just fine. But you will never know what athletic genes may be expressed by interacting with a pro.

If lessons or clinics appeal to you, here are some factors to consider when selecting a pro or program:

- Listening: Do instructors hear what you say? Do they ask questions and think about your answers?
- Feedback quantity: Can be related to listening – or, more precisely, to not listening. Too much feedback, especially for greenhorns, can be confusing, overwhelming, or leading to over-dependence on rules and/or the coach. Opt for someone who regularly stops talking to take a breath.
- Student types: Whom do they now teach? For a coach, one of the greatest achievements is to develop a promising young player into a superstar. As a result, these instructors are enthralled with talented junior athletes, and look askance at someone with grey hair. Or, they might rather deal with an advanced older player, rather than someone totally new to the game. Understand whom they see as their "customer".
  ◦ With respect to an instructor's experience portfolio, men and women who have reached "anecdotage" should not be put off by pros who downplay their chance to excel – nor should they put up with them.
  ◦ Studies have shown that with age, humans don't lose the ability to learn. Tom Vanderbilt explains in

his book, *Beginners*: "As people age, they should not do less, but do more to keep and maintain their abilities.

◦ "But here's another twist: the more learning older adults take on, the faster they seem to learn - the more they become like younger adults. Learning to learn, it seems, is a lifetime sport."[56]

• Empathy: If there's an empathy scale in coaching, rookies may learn more effectively with a pro at the "much empathy" end - that is someone who is patient with their awkwardness, wild moves and unpredictable outcomes. Proficient and expert players, on the other hand, are likely to gravitate to instructors at the "less empathy" end - "...just get to the point..."

• Difficulty perception: Sports are difficult, that's for certain. But a clever instructor can help the beginner by making certain tasks appear easier. It's not rocket science, for example, but by making a golf hole look larger, golfers have an easier time of putting. When they confront a standard hole, they still have an easier time, perhaps because their confidence was boosted by a sense that "hey, this isn't so difficult after all..."[57]

• Reputation: What is the pro known for? Are there good stories and bad? Are these stories believable?

• Student stage of development: Black-visor-wearing Gigi, has some thoughts about selecting a tennis pro for lessons:

"Different pros are needed at different phases of tennis development. Beginners need a pro who can teach the fundamentals, all the shots. Once the player is more advanced, he or she needs a pro who can work on court movement, where to be, and when. Beyond that, you need a pro who can work with your head, and teach you how to put together a point. And, of course, any pro must be compatible with your personality."

Despite the abundance of instructors across the USA, for a given rookie, choices may be limited. In that case, it's helpful to know how to approach a coach and when to cut the cord.

Tips for approaching an instructor:

- Candidly describe your skill level – the pro will recognize it the moment you move, but better to have it fixed as part of your cooperation "agreement". Be skeptical of any coach who tries to rate you up or down.
- Tell the person about any experience you have had with the game such as playing in high school.
- Explain your motivation – Do you want to play with family and friends? Are you looking to become competitive? Is the instructor comfortable with your motives, or does he/she seem to want to nudge you in a different direction?
- Be realistic about how much time you are willing and capable of devoting to the game – and back away from any instructor who quibbles with your scheduling plan.
- Confirm the pro's expectations regarding lesson frequency and timing, class cancellation/late arrival/no show, payment, refunds, substitutes (yours and theirs), venue (e.g., indoor facility as appropriate).

Tips for cutting the cord:

- Begin with the minimum number of lessons possible and agree on criteria for continuing. If you and the coach are *sympatico*, you can always add more.
- Advise the pro of your goals: For example, "...golf well enough to participate in a scramble tournament in two months". Or, "...feel comfortable enough with pickleball to join open play sessions in the fall". If goals aren't reached, you will move on.

Playing

Okay, okay, okay, I've started playing a game, what should I expect?

If you've launched into a sport for the first time, bravo!

Recognize, however, that you will go through a phase that flip-flops between frustration over your rookie skill level and exhilaration about those instances when you perform well.

This is to be expected.

Try the game for a couple of months to see if some of the bumps smooth out. Ask other greenhorns if they are having similar experiences. If you jumped in lesson-free, consider joining a clinic or two.

But, after giving yourself sufficient time to see what's what, recall that you don't have to marry the sport. You two can happily go your separate ways, no (ha, tennis!) strings attached. Figure out what was unsatisfying about the game and identify an alternative without this deficiency.

However, maybe you want to stay married, you just wish for a more blissful union.

A few thoughts on blissfulness

Frequency

The ideal number of times to play a sport is imaginary (!). But the more frequently you play, the more likely you will become good at the game. And the more likely you are good at a game, the more likely you will enjoy it.

It's not a hard-and-fast rule, but, based on the ADAP experience, it is at least a soft-and-slow one.

In general, try to play at least two or three times weekly for six months and then decide whether or not you want to stay married to the game or to divorce it.

This frequency guideline, of course, doesn't apply to the more rigorous sports such as marathons and triathlons. You may find that you can only participate in a "tri" every other month or so, and, in marathons, no more often than every six months.

Easing in

Speaking of marathons and triathlons, it's a good idea to begin with lower levels of competition. For instance, think in terms of 5Ks or half marathons for the former, and sprints for the latter.

Many of the other sports are set up for an easing-in phase. In squash, for instance, the beginner ball bounces friendlier than do balls for more advanced levels. Rowing features novice boats and oars.

Take advantage of these natural progressions.

Inconsistency is a fact of sporting life

Don't be hard on yourself if you inconsistently execute your game of choice. After all, professionals paid to play in the NFL, NBA, LPGA, ATP, MLB, and more decry that they "had a bad day" following some humiliating defeat.

And not just the pros! Take comfort in the fact that amateurs at all levels – beginner, intermediate, advanced – experience lousy outcomes – especially when they cross over to a new endeavor.

Hae

Consider Hae, a 72-year-old golfer who had been a nationally ranked amateur tennis player in her youth.

Her advice to links newcomers? "People need to understand there will be days when you play as if you had never before picked up a club in your life. Need a repeatable swing, consistency."

THE ELIXIR OF SPORT

Develop techniques to give yourself a break on bad days

When your squash shots shoot off in (even more) weird and wonderful directions, or when your pickleball games all seem to go 0-11 on your side, you need a psychic and/or physical boost.

In the mental column, remind yourself that there's more to life than athletics (even though this book is totally enchanted with sports!). Reminisce about some difficult problem you once solved. Contemplate what you will do to celebrate the end of this round/set/game/competition.

In the physical column, when you're between innings, or resting at the end of the pool, or whenever your game reaches a natural break, do what Mom suggested: close your eyes, inhale for a count of five, and then exhale for the same length of time. Subtle stretches and marching in place are also good.

Additionally, identify some options for your sport. Natalya, the one-time Olympic hopeful, had been considering 18 holes of golf to be "obnoxious" but then discovered the nine hole alternative.

If softball's first base stresses you more than it used to, pick up the catcher's face mask.

If drop-in pickleball has become more competitive than you like, start a fun pickleball group.

Discover new aspects of your personality

Originally, Natalya reported, she was not particularly keen on some members of her own gender, due to their tendency for cutting remarks. But she discovered that not all women are divas, and has become good friends with a much larger pool of females.

Remember: Your brain enjoys being unfolded and fluffed on a regular basis

What are some things that enhance playing, aka give your brain a fluff?

First, practice, practice, practice, as the authors of *Road to Automatic* (Chapter 4) recommend.

There are numerous theories that aim to quantify the relationship between practice and expertise. The violinist, for example, should play at least ten million notes before achieving high skill.

How many balls should the pickleball player hit? How many yards should the swimmer swim, or the cyclist pedal?

Second, get used to competition – even competition with yourself.

This is an especially prickly area, as many are put off from a game due to a perception of competition as bullying.

But if you are shy around the 800-pound competition gorilla, perhaps a more forthright willingness to stand up to him would give you and your game a boost.

As bizarre as it may sound, think of competition as a critical step toward self-renewal. Put yourself forth for the challenge. Be "out there" willing to deal with whatever happens. Not talking about specific competitors here, but, rather, the concept itself.

Don't shy from competitive situations, but let them be your reason for playing more, practicing more, focusing more.

If, on the other hand, you are on the hyper-competitive end – maybe you play ping-pong to the death - a more nuanced philosophy would provide lower blood pressure, greater insights, and perhaps more playing partners (hmmm?).

Third, keep in mind that expectations about performance will change as skill increases. For example, when a 3.5 tennis player held a 3.0 rating, the inconsistent elements of the game were the most rudimentary (e.g., hitting lots of high shots, being caught in the wrong part of the court). But that 3.5er has now conquered those inconsistencies, and has replaced them with inconsistent shots that are more finely tuned!

Fourth, be strict about separating practice from play.

At practice, it's fine to think about some critical body part or to experiment with a different move.

For example, the athlete working with a pickleball ball machine may want to try different lateral shuffles and to hit shots with varying wrist action. But during play, the focus is on the ball and only on the ball. Corrections come post-play.

For another example, during a round of golf, it's "game brain," not "practice brain".

On the links, the phenomenon is that golfers take several practice swings for each shot. But the nervous system wants to know, "Well, which is the right swing?" If not that first practice try, is it the second? Or what about the third?

A neurologist will claim that all this swinging confuses the brain, and poses the obvious question: "Which swing does the nervous system use when the golfer is 'really' playing?"

Finally, don't discount chance. The mischievous gods and goddesses of whatever sport one pursues will flip a coin to determine whether one will play well or will stink the place up that day.

While all these challenges can be daunting, remember that there's no substitute for going out there and playing.

"My worst day is a pretty good day…"

Can you say that? Or is your worst day (sports-wise or otherwise) horrendous, miserable, depressing, blah, blah, blah?

This is not to suggest that horrendous, miserable, and depressing things don't happen. Nor that they aren't truly horrendous, miserable, and depressing.

If you can prevent them from occurring, please bottle that! Sometimes, awful days are simply beyond our control.

But it's not the "awful thing" that matters. What matters is <u>how we respond to it.</u>

Can you give yourself just a tiny boost of self-confidence by approaching the "awful thing" as simply a problem to be solved?

Can you strip away any worries about what people will think about your "thing" (e.g., your golf swing "thing") and simply focus on your action, your response, your pulling yourself up?

And what about scoring as a way to focus the mind - rather than as another unfortunate chance to humiliate yourself?

It's basic, but to make a bad day a good one, approach it as such.

THE ELIXIR OF SPORT

Playing is renewing – and it also contributes to long life

Well, despite what the research (Chapter 6) reveals, of course, there's no guarantee that swinging a tennis racquet or kicking a soccer ball (or anything else) will make you live longer.

On the other hand, there's no guarantee that they won't, either.

It's important to remember that the Age-defying Athletes Project has found that there are few other pursuits besides sports that deliver benefits in the here-and-now while also dangling the tantalizing opportunity for a few extra years of life. Good life.

Now that you are finally playing, here-and-now benefits you can expect are fun, friendship, fitness – and love!

- Fun – regain some of that zest you enjoyed as a kid.
- Friendship – games are inherently social – before, during, and afterwards. Athletic pursuit offers limitless conversational fodder. And those who share the joys and sorrows of golf or marathons or cycling have an immediate bond that outranks ties of culture, philosophy, or careers.
- Fitness – minds are sharpened by scoring, strategy, hand-eye coordination and more; bodies become lighter and leaner, strength increases, and unexpected reservoirs of energy emerge.
- Love - Or as some Age-defying Athletes claim, "It's BTS [Better Than Sex]."

Injury

Don't let a setback sideline you permanently.

Ruth (Chapter 8) certainly hadn't expected knee surgery to be on her critical path to the Alpine hiking adventure with her husband. But when it happened, she hung in there, underwent surgery, completed several months of physical therapy, and picked up their preparatory fitness plan where she left off.

That was admirable.

As Age-defying Athletes have reported, however, when they suffer a mishap, they are tempted to rush back in. They resist temptation – and you should, too. Follow the course prescribed by your physician/physical therapist/masseuse/other professional.

But even more important than resisting the temptation to prematurely return to play...

Be smart and practice the Big "P".

Prevention. Prevention. Prevention. Prevent injury from happening in the first place, and avoid all that professional intervention and time off:

- Learn and practice good technique.
- Warm up beforehand, and cool down after.
- Strengthen all your muscles symmetrically (e.g., don't overdevelop your right arm to the detriment of your left), stretch, be kind to your joints.
- And don't overdo it.

"Don't overdo it" is easy to write, but as tough to practice as "Don't rush back in". There's always a tradeoff, for example, between retiring for awhile in order to baby a twingey rotator cuff and just powering through. But, overall, be in it for the long haul, and don't overspend on hurt.

NSC finding

Injury Chapter 8 quotes several statistics from the National Safety Council (NSC) about rates of injury in recreational sports.

In case you were wondering about what activity the NSC ranks as generating the highest rate of injury, the following may surprise you:

For 2022, <u>exercise and exercise equipment</u> was the most harm-prone. The Council reported the statistic that 153 individuals age 65+ per 100,000 population are injured while exercising.[58]

Do gym-goers take bar bells for granted? Are they too blasé about weight room equipment? Who can say? But the statistic is a handy reminder to keep injury in perspective – sometimes it's the most familiar activity that trips people up.

Meaning that you should stay focused, remain in the moment, and practice the Big P!

Brew your own elixir

There is no deterministic way to "navigate the aging process". Rather, you are solely in charge of "climbing the aging ladder" (as Belinda from Chapter 1 opined).

So, as you transition to anecdotage, what will you do, and how will you do it? Will you be proactive, or let the proverbial roof cave in on you?

Athletics are among the greatest companions to have for that walk down life's later path. They provide a resilient structure to the days and generate all those terrific benefits.

That's why the elixir of sport is such a powerful drink – it can help you become the you that you ought to be in later life.

Playing sports is seemingly simplistic, something…well, yes…something you did as a kid. But it kept you young, vital, happy. And it can again.

All you have to do is go out there and play.

Chapter 11
Resources

A few idiosyncratically-selected ingredients to toss into the cauldron as you brew your own elixir

General

Younger Next Year: Live Strong, Fit, and Sexy – until You're 80 and Beyond, Chris Crowley and Henry S. Lodge, https://www.amazon.com/s?k=younger+next+year&crid=3LSHF0GH6LNY&sprefix=younger+next+year%2Caps%2C117&ref=nb_sb_noss_1

What Retirees Want: A holistic View of Life's Third Age, Ken Dychtwald and Robert Morison, https://www.amazon.com/What-Retirees-Want-Holistic-Lifes/dp/1119648084

Beginners: the Joy and transformative Power of Lifelong Learning, Tom Vanderbilt, https://www.amazon.com/Beginners-Transformative-Power-Lifelong-Learning/dp/1524732168

The Ride of Her Life: The True Story of a Woman, her Horse, and their Last-chance Journey across America, Elizabeth Letts, https://www.amazon.com/Ride-Her-Life-Last-Chance-Journey/dp/0525619321

Running

The Run-Walk-Run Method, Jeff Galloway, https://www.amazon.com/Run-Walk-Method%C2%B7/dp/1782550828

Triathlon

Slow Fat Triathlete, Jayne Williams, https://www.amazon.com/s?k=slow+fat+triathlete&crid=2C2XCU6VF0I35&sprefix=slow+fat%2Caps%2C91&ref=nb_sb_ss_fb_1_8_ts-doa-p

Golf

If you want an overview of all courses in your area, Golfnow is helpful, as it provides course information by geography. https://www.golfnow.com/

A lesson option is Operation 36. This innovative program offers instruction at courses all over the world.

The Operation 36 instructional philosophy is to start play at varying distances from the pin – closer for greenest of greenhorns, then farther away as skill develops.

Typically, the early lessons would be 25 yards from the green and focus on short shots and putting.

After a student becomes confident at 25 yards out, he or she moves back to 50 yards from the green, then 100 yards, 150, and, finally, plays from the forward tee. https://operation36.golf/

How to Play Better Golf, Nigel Blenkarn, Jim Christine, Craig DeFoy, Pip Elson, Lawrence Farmer, Lee Fickling, Robin Mann, Tony Moore. Published in 1991 by Ward Lock Limited. Possibly out of print, but may be available at a public library.

Discovering Golf's Innermost Truths: A New Approach to Teaching the Game: A Commentary, John Milton, 2010, https://journals.sagepub.com/doi/abs/10.1260/1747-9541.5.s2.115?download=true&journalCode=spoa

Used clubs are often the most economical way to begin playing the links.

Consider purchasing one or two used clubs at a local thrift shop, Goodwill or Second Swing. The PGA Tour Superstore also offers used clubs. Callawaypreowned.com is an online source, offering several brands.

https://www.2ndswing.com
https://www.pgatoursuperstore.com
https://www.callawaygolfpreowned.com

Tennis

For used tennis racquets, consider one of the online merchants:

Tennis Warehouse https://www.tennis-warehouse.com
Tennis Express https://www.tennisexpress.com

Pickleball

The Dink: Pickleball News and Media,
https://www.thedinkpickleball.com/
For used paddles, check Pickleball Galaxy,
https://www.pickleballgalaxy.com

Swimming

US Masters Swimming is the governing body for swimming, https://www.usms.org/

Governing bodies

A number of sports have overarching associations that develop and manage rules, policies, competitions, and more. Some of these associations may provide information, local opportunities for play, etc.

While the above resources are familiar to or have been recommended to the author, the following listing of governing bodies does not reflect any author knowledge other than what can be gleaned from the web.

Golf

United States Golf Association, https://www.usga.org

Tennis

United States Tennis Association, https://www.usta.com

Bicycling

USA Cycling, https://usacycling.org/, is the governing body for bicycle racing in the United States. It covers road, track, mountain bike, cyclocross, and BMX.

Marathons

Association of International Marathons and Distance Races, https://aims-worldrunning.org/about-aims.html

Triathlons

Combining swimming, running, and bicycling, triathlons in the US have a governing body for "triathlon, as well as duathlon, aquathlon, aquabike, winter triathlon, off-road triathlon and paratriathlon...", https://www.usatriathlon.org/about

International governance is handled by World Triathlon, https://triathlon.org/about

Rowing

US Rowing, https://usrowing.org/

Softball

USA Softball governs softball play in the US, https://www.usasoftball.com/

Yoga

Yoga Alliance, https://www.yogaalliance.org/

Squash

US Squash, https://ussquash.org/

Ping-pong (table tennis)

USA Table Tennis, https://www.usatt.org/

End Notes

[1] *What Retirees Want: A Holistic View of Life's Third Age*, by Ken Dychtwald, Robert Morison, Wiley, 2020.

[2] https://agewave.com/product/what-retirees-want/

[3] Ibid.

[4] Athlete names and other identifying details have been modified throughout this book.

[5] https://www.amazon.com/Toward-Psychology-Being-Abraham-Maslow/dp/0471293091

[6] https://en.wikipedia.org/wiki/Self-actualization#cite_note-ToHM-3

[7] https://eurapa.biomedcentral.com/articles/10.1007/s11556-009-0054-9

[8] Ibid.

[9] https://www.penguinrandomhouse.com/books/574528/the-ride-of-her-life-by-elizabeth-letts/

[10] This is the number of individuals receiving retirement benefits from the US Social Security Administration. Ken Dychtwald and Robert Morison in *What Retirees Want*, peg the total at 68 million.

[11] *Life in Retirement: Pre-Retiree Expectations and Retiree Realities*, Transamerica Center for Retirement Studies, September 2023

[12] Ibid.

[13] Ibid.

[14] Ibid.

[15]

https://www.amazon.com/Run-Walk-Method%C2%B7/dp/1782550828

[16] https://pubmed.ncbi.nlm.nih.gov/15375344/

[17] *Flow: The Psychology of Optimal Experience*; Harper Perennial Modern Classics; 1st edition (July 1, 2008)

[18] *Beginners the joy and transformative power of lifelong learning*, Tom Vanderbilt, Vintage Books, New York, 2021

[19] "The Perpetual Novice: An Undervalued Resource in the Age of Experts," *Mind, Culture and Activity* 4, no. 1 (1997):42-52.

[20] *Mind over Machine, The Power of Human Intuition and Expertise in the Era of the Computer*, Hubert Dreyfus, Stuart Dreyfus; Free Press; Reprint edition (September 12, 1988)

[21] *Beginners the joy and transformative power of lifelong learning*, Tom Vanderbilt, Vintage Books, New York, 2021

[22] https://journals.lww.com/clinicalneurophys/abstract/2004/05000/on_the_road_to_automatic__dynamic_aspects_in_the.2.aspx

[23] Ibid.

[24] Ibid.

[25] *Slow Fat Triathlete*, Jayne Williams, Da Capo Lifelong Books, 2004.

[26] Sport participation and positive development in older persons, *European Review of Aging and Physical Activity* **volume 7**, pages 3–12 (2010)

[27] Ibid.

[28] https://downloads.ctfassets.net/inb32lme5009/7BkRT92AEhVU51EIzXXUHB/37749c3cf976dd10524021b8592636d4/The_Friendship_Report.pdf

[29] "For Some Gen Xers, Skateboarding Is for Life", *Wall Street Journal*, September 5, 2023

[30] https://bjsm.bmj.com/content/51/10/812

[31] https://www.ncbi.nlm.nih.gov/pmc/articles/PMC8391496/

[32] https://www.wellandgood.com/sports-that-increase-life-expectancy/

[33] https://bjsm.bmj.com/content/55/4/206#:~:text=The%20cohort%20of%208124%20US,a%20lower%20risk%20of%20cancer

[34] https://assets-us-01.kc-usercontent.com/c42c7bf4-dca7-00ea-4f2e-373223f80f76/b3eb44f4-d5a2-4501-87ef-6a062771addc/Golf%20and%20Health%20Report.pdf

[35] *Younger Next Year: Live Strong, Fit, and Sexy - Until You're 80 and Beyond*, Chris Crowley, Henry S. Lodge, 2007

[36] Sport participation and positive development in older persons, *European Review of Aging and Physical Activity* **volume 7**, pages 3–12 (2010)

[37] Ibid.

[38] Ibid.

[39] https://eurapa.biomedcentral.com/articles/10.1007/s11556-009-0054-9

[40] https://injuryfacts.nsc.org/home-and-community/safety-topics/sports-and-recreational-injuries/

[41] https://www.sportsmed.org/membership/sports-medicine-update/fall-2023/avoid-a-pickle-know-this-booming-sports-perks-and-pitfalls

[42] https://www.houstonracquetclub.com/

[43] https://www.tennisfame.com/news/2020/original-9-exhibit

[44] https://injuryfacts.nsc.org/home-and-community/safety-topics/sports-and-recreational-injuries/

[45] https://upway.co/

[46] *What Retirees Want: A Holistic View of Life's Third Age*, Wiley; 1st edition (November 24, 2021)

[47] Ibid., Age Wave/Merrill Lynch, *Leisure in Retirement: Beyond the Bucket List*

[48] Ibid.

[49] Ibid.

[50] *Life in Retirement: Pre-Retiree Expectations and Retiree Realities*, Transamerica Center for Retirement Studies, September 2023

[51] Ibid.

[52] Ibid.

[53] Ibid.

[54] https://www.racquetindustryresearch.org/page/research_general

[55] https://www.ngf.org

[56] *Beginners the joy and transformative power of lifelong learning*, Tom Vanderbilt, Vintage Books, 2021.

[57] Adapted from Guillaume Chauvel, et al., "Visual Illusions Can Facilitate Sport Skill Learning," *Psychonomic Bulletin and Review* 22, no. 3 (2015): 717-21.

[58] https://injuryfacts.nsc.org/home-and-community/safety-topics/sports-and-recreational-injuries/

Made in the USA
Columbia, SC
18 February 2025